Turning Black and White into Gray

Turning Black and White into Gray

Mood Disorders: Discovering New Horizons of Understanding and Enlightenment

Sarah Kennedy MFT
and
Keith Conrad

iUniverse, Inc.
Bloomington

Turning Black and White into Gray
Mood Disorders: Discovering New Horizons
of Understanding and Enlightenment

iUniverse books may be ordered through booksellers or by contacting:

iUniverse
1663 Liberty Drive
Bloomington, IN 47403
www.iuniverse.com
1-800-Authors (1-800-288-4677)

ISBN: 978-1-4759-1427-6 (sc)
ISBN: 978-1-4759-1425-2 (e)
ISBN: 978-1-4759-1426-9 (dj)

Library of Congress Control Number: 2012906651

Printed in the United States of America

iUniverse rev. date: 12/07/2012

To my family members and patients, who taught me to understand objectively,

and

Keith, who taught me to understand subjectively. [SK]

To all the people who have had to deal with my ups and downs throughout my childhood and adult life. I hope this book makes it possible for other people to improve the quality of their lives and the lives of their loved ones. [KC]

Contents

Section Two Childhood Neurological Disorders,
   Including Tourette Syndrome

PREFACE

If you are reading this book, you probably just received some devastating news. Very likely a professional informed you that you or your loved one has a neurological problem or mood disorder. It could be attention deficit disorder, bipolar disorder, Tourette syndrome, intermittent rage episodes, obsessive-compulsive disorder, depression, anxiety, or a combination. Many are so similar that it's difficult to determine where one ends and another begins.

Now that you have a name for your symptoms, you may be feeling relief. Or you could be even more confused about what lies ahead.

This information is all new to you, and you may not know where to go from here or how to find help. The future months and years are frightening; you're heading into uncharted territory.

It is our sincere hope that this book will offer you answers and encouragement by providing insight and commonsense tips to comfort, help, and educate you as you explore the many challenges that lie ahead.

Remember to keep things in perspective.

1. Nothing has really changed since the diagnosis was made. Whatever dreams, hopes, and expectations you had before can remain the same. It will likely take a bit more work and understanding to achieve those dreams, but don't give

up. *The diagnosis is only a definition of symptoms.* You can control how much you allow the diagnosis to change how you feel about yourself or other people. It's not what you call it, but what you do about it that really matters.

2. For parents, the diagnosis explains much about the strange behavior you thought may have been caused by your parenting skills. The disorder, not your interactions with your child, caused most of the behavior problems. From now on, you can know that the embarrassing or disruptive behavior is based on a neurological or genetic condition. As you learn more about whatever diagnosis your child has received, you will better understand it and can help educate others about your child's behavior. You'll also start to gain a sense of control, which is likely something new. (This also applies when a spouse or other family member is newly diagnosed.) Education and understanding can provide tremendous assistance to your family while also performing a service to the community. Education is power!

You may not see it now, but there are some benefits associated with mood disorders.

1. If your loved one has a high level of energy, it can often be an asset if properly channeled. You can get the house cleaned, paperwork (or homework) done, or any number of other chores completed. High-energy adults contribute much to the world—they plan and execute with vigor and enthusiasm. These people are often the success stories who achieve the American Dream while the rest of us are sleeping!

2. A common manifestation of Tourette syndrome is obsessive-compulsive disorder (OCD), which is anxiety-induced and often associated with rituals. In OCD, patients suffer from the inability to let go of an idea or thought, without regard to reality. A person who repeatedly checks to see that the door is locked, even though it quite certainly

is, suffers from a manifestation of OCD. Anxiety causes worry about the door being locked and that anxiety is relieved by checking the door *one more time*. A person with OCD feels anxious until the solution to a problem feels just right. Susan writes and rewrites her school paper rather than erasing and correcting a mistake. Carl solves a difficult math problem to an impossibly high standard of perfection. The anxiety from OCD can motivate perfectionists to deliver eloquent speeches, write brilliant poetry, produce beautiful art, or organize meticulous closets "Good enough" is never good enough for them. Standards of perfection inspire goals that greatly benefit society.

3. Attention deficit hyperactivity disorder (ADHD) can include perseveration (persistent repetition of an activity, word, phrase, or movement, such as tapping, wiping, and picking), which makes it appear similar to OCD. Perseveration (a little like perseverance) is the inability to *give up* on an idea or to let it go. For instance, the child who has to shoot one hundred baskets every day, but has no other symptoms of OCD, is probably more likely to fall into the perseveration category. Perseveration is thought to be more closely associated with ADHD. Although patients often have rules about performing a certain activity, the high level of anxiety associated with OCD is generally not seen with perseveration. Also, perseveration generally involves more goal-directed activities, such as shooting a number of baskets or running a number of miles. OCD, in contrast, generally involves anxiety-induced activities without much purpose—activities such as repeated hand washing or lining things up in a particular symmetrical order.

Both OCD and perseveration can be beneficial if channeled creatively. Some speculate that most inventors probably had one of these conditions, as the very act of inventing requires persistence and excessive attention to detail. At the point most people give up, the inventor continues diligently until a new idea is discovered and perfected.

In a somewhat similar way, many athletes are driven to swim one hundred laps every day or to pitch a ball five hundred times to perfect their performance. These actions are more likely to be categorized as perseveration rather than OCD because they are goal-directed. Do you have as much determination and perseverance as these athletes? Few people do. And many who do are champions!

It is extremely important for people with OCD or perseveration to find balance in their lives. Finding a passion provides them with focus. However, without balance in life, there can be a great cost to personal well-being.

One of the most difficult things you'll face is accepting that you or your loved one has a disability, until you realize that everyone has a disability of some kind. Doing the best you can with what life holds for you, no matter how difficult that is, makes all the difference in achieving success.

How can you do this? Continue to read this book. Then read other books. Read articles. Watch films. Go to support group meetings. Talk to people who have been diagnosed with a similar condition. Learn everything you can about the diagnosis. Then learn about other disorders, for there are many areas that overlap among them. The more you know, the better prepared you will be for future problems that may arise. You've taken the first step by reading this book. You're on your way, so keep going, for the journey can be very rewarding.

Introduction

This book is written to explain the different aspects of mood and neurological disorders. It covers attention deficit disorder (with and without hyperactivity), bipolar and unipolar depression, Tourette syndrome, intermittent rage episodes, obsessive-compulsive disorder, and anxiety.

While the above are so closely related that it would be extremely difficult to discuss one without crossing over to the others, the primary focuses of this book are bipolar disorder and Tourette syndrome. The reasons for choosing these two are:

1. There is very limited information available regarding these two topics, especially for the average reader.

2. Bipolar disorder and Tourette syndrome are complex and encompass many of the mood disorders listed above. Discussions of these disorders are included for further interest and understanding..

Turning Black and White Into Gray was written by an adult patient diagnosed with bipolar disorder and his therapist. Both share personal stories that are honest, humorous, sensitive and helpful.

What follows is their journey together, with additional information about related mood disorders. Keith's writing is noted with (KC) while Sarah's is prefaced with (SK).

This inspiring story is written to help you. The honesty will make you think, while the coping skills will offer solutions and hope. Most important, you will realize you are not alone. Now you have the perspectives of the client and the therapist in one book, a book whose time has come.

SECTION ONE
CYCLING DEPRESSION/BIPOLAR DISORDER:
INSIGHTS FROM A PATIENT AND HIS THERAPIST

Chapter One
Cycling Depression/Bipolar Disorder

The Story Begins

Sarah Kennedy started psychotherapy sessions with Keith Conrad in April 2004. At that time, he had depression, anxiety, difficulty concentrating, and trouble controlling his temper. The temper problem was becoming worse and sometimes resulted in "temper tantrums," which scared him and the people around him. He admitted drinking three to six beers every day after work. He felt the beer helped to relax him. This was usually a social event with a few friends who drank with him at his shop.

Keith sought help because his problems were getting worse and were interfering with his career and personal life. Keith's wife was becoming irritated by his late evenings at the shop and "friends" she felt were using him. His work was suffering from his unstructured, chaotic schedule.

Sarah was impressed by Keith's understanding of his weaknesses and problem behaviors. He had undergone many years of prior therapy and knew himself well. However, he had no name for his condition.

Keith's Life

Keith was an only child who was intelligent like his father. He was close to both parents in early childhood. When he was eight, his parents separated, and his world began to crumble. He lived with his mother but enjoyed frequent visits with his father.

Approximately one year after the separation, his father committed suicide. After the suicide, Keith's mother suffered from severe mood swings and a nervous breakdown. She moved Keith to another state to be closer to her family. Keith's stability was rocked and he became a confused, traumatized, lonely boy.

Keith reported that his involvement in a martial arts program as a teenager taught him discipline and provided structure. As an adult, he was involved in a number of short-term relationships.

At age forty-five, Keith had been married for five years and felt his wife was losing patience with his mood swings. His wife's family was somewhat chaotic and outgoing, which was very unlike his. Her parents and four siblings lived close by and celebrated holidays together. She also had two adult children from a previous marriage and shared a close relationship with them. Keith felt he had a good relationship with the members of his wife's family. Before starting therapy, Keith had tried unsuccessfully to reestablish a relationship with his mother, who lived in Nevada (Keith lived in South Dakota).

Sarah's Findings

Keith was pleasant and talkative. He understood how his problems were affecting his life. He was particularly concerned about his excessive anxiety, difficulty sleeping, temper outbursts, and drinking. He was also having negative (dark) thoughts, but he was not suicidal.

Dark thoughts are common in depression. Unipolar depression is usually caused by environmental factors like the death of a loved one, loss of a job, or other personal failure. In unipolar depression, negative thoughts replace positive ones. A sense that nothing is right and something terrible will happen is common. "I'll never get a job because I'm too old" (or "because the economy is failing") are examples of negative thoughts in unipolar depression. These thoughts cause sadness and immobilization with resulting hopelessness and helplessness.

The same pattern is seen in the downward cycle of a patient with bipolar disorder. However, when mania sets in, anxiety can cause negative thoughts to have a "racing" and extremely violent quality. The gruesome thoughts often will not leave the mind. These racing, dark thoughts are terrifying during the day and prevent sleep at night. The patient is fearful that dark thoughts could become reality when he is unable to "escape" them during sleep.

A history of anxiety, racing thoughts, and/or difficulty sleeping is a red flag for considering a diagnosis of a cycling type of depression. Because of its genetic nature, family history is also important. Family members with reports of suicides, "nervous breakdowns", postpartum depression, drug abuse, and/or alcoholism could cause further suspicion of a bipolar diagnosis. This terminology and self-medication could be evidence of a family's tendency toward chemical imbalance associated with a genetic form of depression.

Keith tested highly positive for attention deficit hyperactivity disorder (ADHD) and mild depression. Sarah suspected a cycling type of depression (possibly bipolar disorder) because of Keith's mood swings, anxiety, dark thoughts, sleep problems, and temper tantrums. She was further suspicious because of his father's suicide and mother's nervous breakdown. She recommended psychiatric evaluation for formal diagnostic evaluation of Keith's condition and treatment of his condition.. Keith was unable to schedule an appointment with a psychiatrist for six weeks. He chose to see his primary medical doctor for immediate treatment of his anxiety symptoms and then transfer his care to a psychiatric facility as soon as possible.

In the first two weeks, Keith saw his medical doctor for an emergency appointment. The doctor wrote him a prescription for an antianxiety medication, (Xanax). This was to help him manage anxiety and temper outbursts until he could see the psychiatric specialist. Xanax is effective for occasional or short-term use, but is potentially highly addictive. While on Xanax, Keith's anxiety decreased and his temper outbursts were controlled. However, it was likely that the psychiatric specialist would prescribe a different long-term medication.

When Keith was seen by the psychiatric specialist, his Xanax was decreased and then discontinued. Keith was started on Prozac, which is a selective serotonin reuptake inhibitor (SSRI) commonly used to treat depression. Initially, Keith did extremely well on Prozac. He said he had "never felt so good; this was his first window of feeling normal." He was happy, relaxed, and could sleep. His dark thoughts were gone and he had an optimistic attitude. Unfortunately, he developed side effects that forced him to discontinue the medication.

He was then changed to Wellbutrin. This is a medication that is effective in treating both depression and attention deficit disorder. The psychiatric specialist hoped it would help with both problems. On Wellbutrin, Keith's concentration improved and he could perform his job duties better. He felt like raging but could talk himself out of his anger and avoid temper outbursts. Wellbutrin is not as sedating as Prozac. Therefore, Keith was given a small quantity of Xanax to help him relax and sleep. This was carefully monitored.

Bipolar disorder is usually treated most effectively with a mood stabilizer. Mood stabilizers are the "big guns" of psychotropic medications and are generally prescribed and monitored by psychiatrists. Mood stabilizers include lithium and antiseizure medications like Depakote, Lamictal, and Tegretol. Primary medical doctors and psychiatric physician assistants are comfortable prescribing antidepressants and antianxiety medications. However, when a mood stabilizer is necessary, referral to a psychiatrist is indicated.

Keith reported that medications were always very effective on him and he usually required only a minimal dose. It made sense that Wellbutrin and Xanax would be adequate to treat his symptoms and psychiatric evaluation could be postponed. Keith agreed to follow up in Sarah's office often to work on relationship problems and to continue on his current medications.

Keith was stable for four months. His dark thoughts were controlled and he was able to reason with people; he was rebuilding his relationships and business. He had less anxiety and could talk himself out of temper outbursts.

Keith continued weekly therapy sessions to work on relationship issues. Hypnotherapy helped with his anxiety and sleep difficulties.

All was well from April until mid-August, when Keith and his wife came to see Sarah for couples' therapy. In the couples' session, Sarah noticed that Keith was different. He thought he could "do anything" in his printing business. He was not sleeping while working long hours. It seemed there was nothing he could not accomplish. Day and night he worked endless hours to finish printing jobs. His wife was concerned, but Keith had a grandiose feeling of accomplishment. Sarah noted this questionable manic episode.

Keith returned a few days later, more stable and relaxed. He reported he was sleeping and no longer spending long hours at his job. The following week in a couples' session, Keith and his wife were doing well.

When seen alone the next week, Keith was depressed and suicidal. His optimism had been replaced by a negative attitude. Much of the work he had finished while manic was returned to him with complaints about mistakes and omissions. He was frustrated having to correct these jobs. He said he felt like he was "chasing his tail." He reviewed his life and verbally beat himself up for past failures. It was the first time Sarah had a hard time following Keith's logic.

Sarah felt she had seen Keith go from mania into the depths of depression in a very short time. She was very worried about Keith and instructed him to schedule an appointment with a psychiatrist for diagnosis and treatment of probable bipolar disorder. He was further advised to contact his psychiatric specialist. He promised to check in with Sarah daily and to call immediately if his condition worsened. Keith's wife was called and informed about his condition.

Keith saw the psychiatrist, who confirmed the diagnosis of bipolar disorder. The psychiatrist prescribed a mood stabilizer and Keith gradually improved.

Sarah continued to see Keith regularly and to coordinate his care with the psychiatrist when indicated. Through their work together, Keith's understanding of his condition improved and his outcome was excellent.

[SK]

I have often thought that bipolar is the cruelest of all mood disorders because of the way patients experience windows of "normal" (whatever that is). These windows can last days, weeks, months, or longer. When the patient subsequently enters a manic or depressed state, there is great confusion. Where did "normal" go and how can it return? Was it a dietary or sleep change, or something environmental? This search for the window of "normal" is frustrating. It is difficult to understand and accept the chemical nature of the mood changes. There is nothing that can be done to find this elusive "normal". It is a chemical change in the brain.

People in a manic state see life with a greater intensity than most of us, and that can be both a blessing and a curse. Brilliant minds produce creativity that lends itself well to artistic genius. A combination of grandiose ideas, racing thoughts and sleepless nights often become ideal for converting brilliance into greatness. With treatment some passion is lost. The intensity with which patients experience life and express themselves through art, poetry, music and writing can be decreased. Sometimes bipolar patients exchange genius for mediocrity; sometimes they must in order to survive.

The list of famous people with characteristics of bipolar disorder is fairly long. While we can't go back in history to diagnose these creative geniuses, there's much evidence to indicate that composers Amadeus Mozart and Ludwig van Beethoven, poet Edgar Allan Poe, author Ernest Hemingway, artist Vincent van Gogh, actresses Patty Duke and Carrie Fisher, singer Judy Garland, entertainer Marilyn

Monroe, and musician Kurt Cobain had characteristics of bipolar disorder.

The list above offers only some of the people whose names would be recognized. Consider the great contributions society has received from people coping with their bipolar conditions. While we benefit from their gifts, many have paid a high price—lived lives of anxiety, loneliness or sadness that sometimes led to suicide. When treated, the highs aren't as high anymore, but the lows aren't as low either. Some passion is replaced by predictability and stability. Adults who are used to the productive highs are often reluctant to lose them by taking medication. They have learned to compensate. They find the newly-medicated versions of themselves to be dull and mediocre.

When considering proper treatment, each patient must make a careful decision on the basis of this double-edged sword and the recommendations of the treating psychiatrist.

Mild bipolar disorder is called cyclothymia. Many people with cyclothymia are not aware they have a form of the disorder and may just believe they have mood swings. "Cycling depression" is a label that can be used for patients who fall somewhere within the bipolar spectrum. The term "bipolar disorder" can be frightening to patients and most do not understand what "cyclothymia" means. "Cycling depression" is a descriptive term that is nonthreatening.

Sarah's Clinical Background:
I had a lot of personal and professional experience with pathological patients. I had raised a child with many problems including Tourette syndrome, ADHD, dyslexia and bipolar disorder. I often wondered what caused the unusual behavior I observed. I had good insight from a parent's point of view.

In the early years of my clinical practice in California, I learned how ADHD, Tourette syndrome, bipolar disorder, autism, OCD, and other mood and neurological disorders adversely affected siblings, parents, and patients.

Over the years, the number of patients with bipolar disorder increased. I observed the tragic effects as families and patients tried to cope with this illness and I helped in whatever ways I could. There was limited information available but I continued to be fascinated by the challenge and the frustrating way it caused so much chaos. It seemed there was little understanding of something that was becoming so common. I wanted to educate the public and help the troubled people who suffered from this condition. At that time, I had little knowledge of a patient's subjective feelings. How did it feel to be the person with the disorder?

When I relocated my practice to South Dakota, I would learn about that from a bipolar patient who had excellent insight and a unique ability to express it.

Perhaps because of the change of seasons and a prevalence of seasonal affective disorder (SAD), I found bipolar disorder to be more common in the Midwest than in California. Many patients with the disorder began to surface in South Dakota. SAD is associated with cycling depression or bipolar disorder. As the weather becomes dark and dreary in the winter months, depression increases for the bipolar patient. A sunny climate improves bipolar symptoms and many people with SAD purchase sunlamps to help improve their moods through the long winter months. These sunlamps are an electrical substitute for Mother Nature and help alleviate the darkness of winter.

It is possible that bipolar disorder is the most underdiagnosed and undertreated psychological disorder in the United States. Untreated bipolar disorder can lead to family problems, drug addiction, alcoholism, crimes, and suicides.

New Kind of Depression

Over the past few years, a new kind of depression has emerged in the United States. It is a cycling type of depression that is both genetic and biochemical. It responds best to mood stabilizers rather than the standard antidepressants (mainly selective serotonin reuptake inhibitors, or SSRIs) that have been used for generations to treat environmentally-induced unipolar depression.

I've been a practicing counselor since 1994 and watched this new type of depression become more common. The following is a list of experiences afflicted patients have described.

1. Episodes of problems with sleep.

2. Problems with out-of-control spending.

3. Family (or personal) history of alcoholism or drug abuse.

4. Family (or personal) history of nervous breakdowns.

5. Family (or personal) history of postpartum depression.

6. Road rage, rage episodes, or family members with rage episodes.

7. Family history of suicide.

8. Personal suicide attempt(s).

9. Seasonal affective disorder.

10. Racing thoughts.

11. Self-mutilation (cutting, eraser burning, head banging, etc.).

12. Promiscuity.

13. Symptoms began or became severe in teen years.

It is extremely important as a clinician to take a thorough and careful patient and family history if bipolar illness is suspected. Many of the above criteria are often present.

It is also important to note that many of these patients appear to be functionally normal or above normal, making it even more important to take a careful history.

Initial Treatment

The bipolar patient frequently presents in a manic state and is therefore having severe difficulty with anxiety and lack of sleep. Many times, well-meaning clinicians prescribe SSRIs before considering a mood stabilizer when the patient clearly has signs of bipolar disorder. SSRIs are the class of drugs, including Prozac, Luvox, Paxil, Zoloft, Lexapro, and Celexa, that generally regulate levels of serotonin in the brain.

Starting with SSRIs can be time-consuming and frustrating for patients who are already suffering from an illness that is debilitating to their professional and personal lives. Many SSRIs require up to a month to become effective. Therefore, it can take one or two months to determine whether a medication is effective. If ineffective, it is then changed to another SSRI, which can take another month or two to evaluate. Thus, it often takes months of trying different SSRIs before determining none is going to work and something different should be tried. By that time, the patient is often extremely frustrated and even more depressed than before. Hospitalization is sometimes required at this stage.

It is important for medical professionals to become familiar with the symptoms of cycling depression so the proper treatment with a mood stabilizer can commence in a timely manner. A careful history can prevent potential delays. with ineffective medications. Knowledge about the differences between unipolar and bipolar depression is invaluable for all medical professionals. This knowledge can help practitioners avoid tremendous expense as well as potentially painful experiences for patients and their families.

A large percentage of untreated bipolar patients commit suicide. Many of these frustrated patients have turned to self-medication with alcohol or street drugs in an effort to alleviate their symptoms. It is a clinical obligation to treat these patients correctly to prevent this potential tragedy. A proper diagnosis will reduce the costs associated with unnecessary doctor visits, medication changes, and potential hospital stays, while decreasing mortality rates.

In the recent past, there has been an increase in the abuse of prescription drugs. Many times, patients who cannot sleep take large quantities of anti-anxiety or sleeping pills. Most of these are in the classification of benzodiazepines, which are effective when monitored carefully but tend to be habit-forming. Common benzodiazepines include Xanax, Valium and Ativan. Many sleeping pills are also in the benzodiazepine category. These medications are valuable in the treatment of a number of conditions. However, they are addictive and must be monitored carefully to prevent abuse.

My theory is that when a bipolar patient is in a down swing, her metabolism slows down and less medication is needed. In this down cycle, she may perceive that she is overmedicated and cut back on the dose. When she then enters a manic phase, everything speeds up, including perhaps metabolism. Her body metabolizes medication faster and she may believe she requires more to feel the same effects as before. On the prior dose of benzodiazepines, she is anxious and sleep is difficult. She takes a higher dose of medication, not realizing she is overdosing. When this increased dose fails to work, she may add alcohol searching for a relaxing effect. She continues to take more medication until she feels the same degree of relaxation as before, never realizing she has taken a dangerously high (perhaps lethal) dose.

Bipolar patients require a proper consistent medication regimen that is carefully monitored by a psychiatrist. Because of the inconsistent nature of bipolar illness, there is a tendency for substance abuse. A responsible psychiatrist can help to prevent this tragedy.

A Theory about Why Depression Is on the Increase
The people who immigrated to the United States were disconnected at home in some way. The happy people stayed in their homeland. Those who were dissatisfied with life (depressed) came to America, and those who were adventurous and wanted to start a new life (ADHD) came to America. Therefore, the United States became a land of adventurers and depressed people—all looking for a better life.

ADHD is known to have a genetic basis, which is a theory for its rise in numbers over the years. Likewise, cycling depression is genetic. Over the generations, depressed people married and had children, resulting in a genetically depressed people. Thus, the depressed people we see today have an increased likelihood of suffering from genetic cycling depression rather than the environmentally-induced type identified more frequently in the past.

[KC]

I have read that short cycling depression is very hard to treat, but I think you have to remember that a person has two cycles—an internal cycle and an external cycle. The external cycle is prompted by stress, change, weather, and day-to-day confrontations, while the internal cycle just makes each one of these external prompts more intense.

During the low points of my yearly cycling (April and October tend to be my low points), if I have a stressor, I seem to become more angry than euphoric. Then it is very difficult to live with me. I feel the difficulty comes from me being depressed, and my body is burning up the medication because of my anger. As things become more hopeless, I look to self-medicate with adrenaline. At least that's what I think is going on, because during these low points, I seem to become very irritable. The stress dumps me full of adrenaline, and my body enters a fight-or-flight mode.

Like many people with bipolar disorder, I like to drink alcohol. I notice my drinking cycles increase during the spring and fall. I want to drink two or three beers—sometimes more—every night during these low periods. Being aware of this pattern is a way for health care professionals and others to understand the low points and the behaviors connected with them.

Mania versus Depression

One thing to note here concerns a missed diagnosis—the time when people say, "Well, I think he is going into a manic state." And, perhaps for the short term, I am a bit manic. But in the longer term, I'm definitely in a state of despair and depression. When people study the statistics of suicide and attempted suicide, I wonder if any reference is made to whether the people studied were in a low cycle or not.

There is a statement that helps me, and may help others suffering from mood disorders too: "Always prepare for the worst, but expect the best." It's a kind of a strange thing. In most cases, if there happens to be a problem, I'm going to always expect the worst. It's always going to be, "Oh, my God, the letter is lost," or "the keys are lost," or "somebody stole my wallet." It's an unusual defense mechanism that comes into play. But I also expect the best. It's a two-sided coin.

When I expect the best, I expect perfection, which is impossible. At least people tell me perfection is impossible, but I still strive for it in some instances.

And that brings me to the duality involved in my quest for expecting the best—I always seem to focus on the worst-case scenario. If one little thing does not go my way, it's the end of the world.

People tell me I have a pessimistic attitude, and while that may be true, I think it's more that I'm suffering from a cycling disorder that keeps me in the lower reaches of a swing much more than in a manic state.

On the other hand, those who suffer unipolar depression simply go down, feel sad, cry, and show very little or no emotion. As a bipolar person, when I feel depressed, I can actually get nervous and aggressive. In my case, with short cycling, I can cycle by the hour, and if the right stressor hits me, I go down.

Preparing for the Worst, Expecting the Best

Preparing for the worst and expecting the best presents a problem in that it makes perfect sense to me, but the people I live and interact with each day find it extremely unnerving. If you're a family member of a person with mood swings, you probably know what I'm talking about.

Perhaps the best way to describe preparing for the worst and expecting the best is the example of the glass being half full or half empty. To us, the glass is half full, but be careful because the damn thing can spill. We expect it to be full; it's actually half empty and half full; and we have to be careful because we might kick it over.

That thinking is unnerving for people who try to live in a positive mind-set. And, really, if you understand the fact that the moods that swing pretty much stay low, it makes sense that pessimism is a norm. I call it pessimism, but my wife calls it drama, drama, drama. And, yes, I can be dramatic at times.

I recall a time when both of us had been working extremely long hours in the business, and we lost an envelope that held a deposit for the bank. We thought the envelope possibly got put in with a bunch of letters for the mailbox. Well, I did not take that possibility in a positive sense, which really was upsetting for my wife. She found the deposit envelope. But, of course for me, "It's in the trash. Now what are we going to do? We're going to have to call the people and tell them we lost the checks. Yada yada …"

It's like the glass being half empty and half full. In many ways, my perspective was real. That's one example that shows a bipolar can be an extreme realist.

If you say the glass is half empty, that's your conclusion. If you say the glass is half full, that is your conclusion. If we listen to our internal coach, we understand that to get positive results, we must see the glass as half full. But to see it both ways can be helpful.

As I look back over my life, how I saw the glass half empty had a way of holding me back. When I decided the glass was half full, I pressed on, trying to fill it up. When I saw it was half empty, I looked for ways to conserve what there was. Like so many people who are busy going up and down, I had a hard time moving forward. Many people are stuck between the positivity and negativity of life.

When I question whether it's bad to see the glass half empty or half full, I recognize the bad thing is that thinking can hold you back or cause you to spend too much time worrying, analyzing, or trying to understand. That, in turn, causes you to be inconsistent with how you see things, how you react, and how you communicate with family members or associates.

Family members who deal with the mood swings of a person who has black-and-white thinking should consider redirecting that person when the negativity becomes too much. We are most likely trying to solve a problem, and all the negative possibilities rush into our heads first. When we're expressing negativity, we're really reflecting the onslaught of negative thoughts we're having. That doesn't mean we are truly negative, and we know that, but you may not. We can get so caught up in the process that we lose track of time and get stuck in a very bad place. So you can help by bringing us out of our thoughts and suggesting other options.

[SK]

I often hear family members of bipolar patients refer to "Mary's World" or "Joe-Land," which is a dark place where patients are striving for perfection and beauty. Loved ones describe "walking on eggshells" in order to keep things on an even keel. The person inside the other world is suffering greatly, striving for perfection—an impossible achievement.

People dealing with bipolar disorder are among the most creative and brilliant minds on the planet. They bring many gifts to society, yet can frustrate both themselves and those around them. The sooner we properly diagnose bipolar disorder, the sooner these people can move forward in life. Wasting months trying medications that aren't effective does no one any good.

One of the interesting aspects of having bipolar disorder is the ability to see two perspectives—opposite perspectives—and see the benefit of each. To the family member, the perspectives appear extreme or dramatic, and indeed they can be, but the bipolar patient doesn't see that. Instead, he or she may first be bombarded with the negative, and may reflect on that before the positive comes to light.

As you continue to read each of our perspectives, we know you'll gain a better understanding of what it's like when your days are all about turning black and white into gray.

Bipolar Triggers

There are many common bipolar triggers. If you are familiar with these triggers, you can often learn to help yourself to prevent major mood swings. Some of the personal and most preventable triggers are:

1. *Not having a consistent sleep schedule.* It is extremely important for people with bipolar disorder to get enough sleep.

2. *Missing meals or eating a diet that is not healthy.* It is also extremely important to eat a diet high in protein, with frequent snacks. Ideally, the bipolar should eat six times a day: three light meals and three snacks.

3. *Stopping or starting medicine for depression or another illness.* It is important to remember that mood stabilizers are the drugs of choice for treatment of bipolar disorder. Many antidepressants make the disorder worse over time.

4. *Misusing alcohol or drugs.* Substance abuse doesn't help and definitely hurts.

5. *Thyroid or other health problems.* It is important to have frequent medical exams and blood work to rule out any health problems that may arise or be concurrent with bipolar disorder. Thyroid disorder is one of the most common. Low thyroid function (hypothyroidism) or high thyroid function (hyperthyroidism) can mimic the depression or mania associated with bipolar illness. It is important to have thyroid function checked regularly over the course of treatment.

6. *Seasonal changes* can affect the severity of bipolar. Fall and spring are the most common times of year for weather-related triggers to occur. Most people with bipolar disorder have some kind of depression the entire winter season in frigid climates. These types of seasonal problems are much less common (or nonexistent) in warmer climates, where the weather is warmer and more stable.

7. *Holidays* can cause tremendous stress, resulting in anxiety and cycling. Of course, any kind of stress, including problems with family or friend, or at work, can also create stress and anxiety, which will result in cycling episodes.

8. *The death of a loved one*, which creates the most stress of all, creates the greatest trigger and thus the greatest potential for mood swings.

It is extremely important to become aware of your triggers and possible triggers. They can be used to track your feelings and to track your patterns.

Talk with family and friends about your patterns. Your loved ones can help you identify and deal with your patterns.

Don't be afraid to ask for help. Most people are more than willing to help you if they know what you need.

Chapter Two
Self-Medication

[KC]

I said in the last chapter that often bipolars and people with other mood disorders like to drink. I did. A lot of times I was surrounded by some of my so-called friends and we'd drink. It became a pattern, and a pattern meant consistency.

The pattern took one of two tracks. In the first, I'd drink. The alcohol took effect. I would begin to ruminate on how crappy my day was. My friends would drink with me. The alcohol took effect. They would begin to ruminate on how crappy their days were.

In the second pattern, I'd drink. The alcohol took effect. I would become jovial and fun and inspirational to my friends as I listened to their problems and even offered some solutions. In retrospect, I doubt we ever solved any of our problems by discussing them through the veil of alcohol. Instead, we just sat around together, ruminated, and wasted time.

After I was married and clearly saw the problems my drinking caused, I decided not to drink at work any longer. My friends resented this decision and, with their black-and-white thinking, blamed it on my wife.

Now that I'm better, I look back and see that my friends helped me stay on an unhealthy path. We didn't change. Why would we? We were used to being angry and negative, and we reinforced each other's reality.

Alcohol and Medication

Some people think of alcohol as hard liquor only, but wine and beer are alcohol too. What I found is that you can't mix alcohol and medication. The two are not a good combination. Prior to medication, I handled the alcohol differently. But with medication, I began making errors at work. After drinking beer the night before, I wasn't as alert the following day, although I did not realize this.

I was upset with my friends for blaming my wife that I didn't want to drink beer on work evenings. I told them it wasn't her, but instead it was the errors I was making that caused me to make the decision. Now as I reflect on that incident, I have a better understanding of my friends' reactions. When I said no to drinking, I created a sudden change in their routine. I wasn't consistent anymore.

The inconsistency with Keith didn't set well. They were used to having drinks with Keith, ruminating about problems, and then doing nothing to solve those problems. When I said no to alcohol, in essence I was saying, "I'm solving my own problem, why don't you?"

Motivation for Drinking

If I haven't been clear so far, I want to make sure you understand I owned the business—I wasn't an employee drinking at work. I was the boss. Usually I worked late and only drank after business hours.

Why would I drink? At times it was at the end of the day. I usually had a lot of anxiety about what I didn't get done and what I was supposed to do, or seeing an employee who wasn't giving 110 percent.

A business consultant told me once that all I could expect from an employee was about 60 percent, and if I got that, an employee was top notch. Well, I drive myself 110 percent, so I became frustrated when I saw employees doing less. As soon as everyone left, I drank, so that made me a closet drinker more or less.

I wasn't a binge drinker. I maybe got really, totally drunk once or twice a year, usually at banquets when I drank hard liquor. The alcohol seemed to lower my anxiety level.

What's also interesting is the alcohol disconnected my stops or control mechanisms that kept me from either acting like an idiot or becoming extremely agitated.

Drinking Alone

Sometimes when I was alone, I'd listen to old music, the music that soothes the savage beast. Without the music, I became more infuriated. I actually wanted people to come around after I had consumed three or four beers, because that was the point when we could talk about problems.

Even when I was out drinking with my friends, I'd eventually go home. Before I got married, I was alone when I got home, so I listened to music and maybe drank some more. After I got married, I'd go home and dump all my problems on my wife—remember, all the stops were out.

To show how I'd let my wife have it, here's something that happened. We got a refund. She wanted to give her son some money (she had her reasons, but I didn't want to hear them). Her son was twenty-four years old and had a good job at the time. Immediately my control mechanism went totally awry and I started spewing out, "Can we afford it? Are you crazy?" And then I hit way below the belt and dragged her ex-husband into it.

If I looked at things objectively, her ex-husband did contribute his fair share and he gave a lot of money for his children before they became adults, so I shouldn't belittle the man for being bitter. But I became defensive about how to use our refund and I wanted her ex-husband to pay. I asked, "What does he pay?" Then I added, "You know you guys always protect him and leave me swinging in the wind."

Unfortunately, with alcohol, this negative attitude always seems to be the pattern.

Do I recommend drinking? You can tell from what I've already said that I don't think it's a good idea, but I also think that a person can have a couple of social drinks if you make sure you have a full stomach first. Of course, other factors must be considered, including whether you personally have an alcohol issue. Each case needs individual consideration.

Change Brings Change

When I started therapy, took my medication, and changed my drinking habits, I experienced another change. My old buddies didn't want to hang out with me so much anymore. They are people who are afraid of change. Like most other humans, they need consistency and a sense of belonging. Drinking did that for them—offered a sense of belonging, a sense of camaraderie.

What is the solution? Do you get rid of the friends, end friendships you've had for many years? I can't answer for you, but one thing I found was that I was feeling a great deal of anger when I was in that drinking mode. Anger is probably one of the most damaging emotions you can have, because it's like the chicken and egg question—which came first? When you are stressed, you become angry, and anger cranks up the stressors. It's a vicious cycle.

I read an article about anger and the author said that if you want to get rid of your anger, and if you truly want to control your anger, then you have to be careful about who you pick for friends. Why? Many people are angry at other people. If you pick angry people to be your friends, you connect on that level.

That's what happened when my old friends and I would drink together. As the alcohol took the stops out, we could all be angry together. Examine your own circle of friends. Do you sit around being angry together? I looked at my personal relationships and saw that for the most part, on my side, they all lasted about two years. Healthy relationships typically last a lot longer than that. You need to ask yourself, "Are these people really nurturing me, or are they adding to my problems?" If they're adding to your problems, you probably need to change your relationship with them.

[SK]

Mood Disorders/Bipolar Disorder and Self-Medication

Because there's a tendency for most people with mood disorders to self-medicate with substances, including alcohol, marijuana and illegal street drugs, each case must be considered on an individual basis. Untreated adult bipolar patients tend to find these substances and to abuse them until proper treatment is found. Because of its relaxing effects, marijuana is a particularly popular form of self-medication for bipolar disorder. Marijuana often helps bipolar patients to sleep, and reduces their anxiety significantly, which often decreases the severity of a manic episode. ADHD patients often find a form of methamphetamine or cocaine because these are stimulants which improve the focus of ADHD patients.

Until mood disorders are more widely recognized and treated, the frequent use of illegal drugs and alcohol will be common forms of self-treatment for the symptoms of these disorders. Unfortunately, the symptoms are often worsened by these substances over the long term, while the proper medications abate the symptoms. It's sad that these patients struggle for so many years as they search for an answer to the confusing and frustrating symptoms from which they suffer

Often people with psychological differences spend years searching for the norm. Bipolar patients search for the normal state of being between manic and depressed states. Obsessive-compulsive patients wonder how much the average person worries about symmetry and balance, promptness, or intrusive thoughts. People with phobias wonder how they can overcome exaggerated unrealistic fears of targeted objects.

Keith had dealt with mood swings and ADHD his entire adult life and had undergone many years of personal counseling. Through psychotherapy and education, he had acquired excellent insight regarding his symptoms. However, he had not yet identified what was happening to him because he had no diagnosis.

It's easy to observe other people and tell them what they're doing wrong. If you see loved ones drinking, you can see a behavior change (whether to an angry or cheerful mood). However, alcohol has changed their brain chemistry, making it difficult for intoxicated people to recognize the extent of difference in their behavior.

With hard work, reflection, and introspection, a bipolar patient can learn the adverse effects of alcohol and make a decision to stop drinking alcohol. When that happens, this person is going to need your support and reinforcement. Make sure you're ready to offer assistance. In severe cases of alcoholism, hospitalization may be required for treatment.

Chapter Three
Variety

[KC]

Cycling depression used to be called manic-depressive disorder. I want to talk about what the manic state is like.

On one occasion, I had been in a manic state for three days. The good news was that it had been almost a year since I had been that way. What set it off was a confrontation with a friend who insulted my wife. All of a sudden, other things which I should have let go of or forgotten seemed to well up. What's interesting is it seems that in a manic mind (or at least in my mind), a tremendous amount of negative energy can get stored. So can a lot of positive energy. It just seems that the positive energy is a little harder to access. Is that all attributable to bipolar disorder, or is some part of it ritual and habit? I'm not sure we know, but either way, it's real. And during that three-day manic state, I felt angry for all three days.

[SK]

Degrees of Manic States

There are different degrees of manic states. It has been theorized that the longer the period between episodes, the more severe the manic episode will be. However, in the case of Keith and with many other bipolar patients, there were shorter (milder) cycles superimposed upon the longer (more severe) cycles. Keith was having weekly, sometimes daily, cycles of less severity that were part of his semiannual (often spring and fall seasons) longer, severe cycles. A short cycle in the middle of summer would likely be of less intensity than one at the end of October, when a longer seasonal cycle was present.

A number of bipolar patients report having experienced primarily short cycles, and others describe longer periods between mood swings. Patients who have short cycles can be difficult to medicate because of the ever-changing nature of this illness. One hour they may be manic, with a high metabolism that requires a high dose of medication for control. The following hour they could sink to a depressed state with decreased metabolism, causing a feeling of being overmedicated. It is important for short-cycling patients to maintain regular diets and consistent sleep patterns. Prescribed medications must be administered on a regular time schedule. For these patients, changes in structure will almost always cause problems, and consistency must be maintained, *no matter how they feel*.

Sometimes people with longer cycles believe they no longer need medication, and it can be difficult to argue otherwise. I had a patient who had a normal cycle that lasted more than nine years. With the guidance and agreement of his psychiatrist, he made the decision to discontinue his medication. However, when he became manic, he went into a rage state that caused a tremendous amount of damage and was personally devastating.

It is easy to understand why it is often difficult to manage the medication of these patients, or to even convince them of the necessity of taking it. This decision belongs to each patient and must be made based upon the severity of the disorder and other factors determined by the patient and psychiatrist.

[KC]

Medication

One of the reasons it is really hard for me to stay on my medication is the fact that prior to taking the medications, being manic actually enhanced my work mode. I could work twenty hours a day. I was clear-thinking. I could even solve problems at an almost breathtaking speed.

Since beginning mood stabilizers, antianxiety medications, and antidepressants, I find the manic states drain me. Just like any time I was in a manic state but less severe than before medication, I still spew the negative energy out, as if I were dumping toxic waste. Unfortunately, during one of my manic states, I almost brought the members of my family to the point of having nervous breakdowns.

This spewing is a strange thing. You seem to want to get the negative out of your system, and then you look at the effect you're having on the people you love. At first, you almost want them to hurt like you hurt—you want them to feel bad. Then you think, "Oh, I can think. I can do things." And you want to help the one you just hurt. You begin the manic state with an I-don't-care attitude because your whole world is focused on you. Later, you're sorry for letting others feel your anger.

I talked in the last chapter about being alone and drinking. Mania creates isolation, or at least leads to becoming isolated.

Once the manic state starts, you cannot stop it. So it's imperative to understand the triggers in order to stop the rituals that bring mania on. Once mania starts, your metabolism becomes so accelerated that the medication gets used up quickly, which impacts your chemical balance.

When I was in a manic state, I would have to spew on people, dump toxic waste, or seek adrenaline. When I sought adrenaline, I had to push myself into a form of actual frenzy or life-threatening consequence. Then it seemed like a switch was tripped and the adrenaline flowed—it was dangerous, extremely dangerous. I've noticed that now my manic states are driven by my anxiety.

Of course one should never alter medication without first consulting with the doctor. My doctor and I discovered that a change in medication during a manic state helped me. When I increased the dosage of the antianxiety medication, the manic state came down much more effectively than if I took the mood stabilizer alone. What I was doing was hitting the trigger, stopping the trigger, stopping the anxiety, and then beginning to wind down the mania.

An interesting and profound discovery I made regarding the adrenaline and antianxiety medication taken in the manic state is that the adrenaline flow no longer seemed to do its job the way it had done before. In fact, the adrenaline became toxic, as it does for the average person.

If you can stop the anxiety, you can lower the intensity of the manic state. Taking antianxiety medication in the manic state can slow the system down so that what's left of the other medications can then work.

For me, it's more effective to take the antianxiety medications three times a day—morning, noon, and night. In the beginning, I had some issues with the medication keeping me awake at night, but that gradually subsided.

People with cycling depression have to learn to function in the manic state without getting lethargic and dipping down. Is it possible to create a positive manic state? I think so. Find something like competitive sports or even video games to channel the energy. The important thing to take away from this is that if you can stop the anxiety, you can slow the mania down, and possibly even stop it.

[SK]

One of the reasons for adrenaline-seeking behavior appears to be to burn up the extra energy present during a manic state. Once the energy is burned up, there is an almost opposite, sometimes relieving and calming effect, such as that which is present in the treatment of ADHD patients with stimulant medications.

The belief that the manic state is productive is common with many bipolar patients. But at what price? They *think* they are doing well; however, they often make mistakes because of the periods of sleep deprivation. In the short-term, they do well. However, often in the larger picture, they suffer because of other health problems and business and personal mistakes.

Chapter Four
Cycles

[KC]

We talked about short-cycling bipolar depression earlier. I short cycle, normally. I mean I can be up and down, up and down through the day. This is very hard to treat because when I'm up, I am burning up my medication like crazy. I burn it up, it's gone, and I plummet down. Some things that cause me to short cycle are day-to-day stresses, being very busy, or skipping a meal. If stress is the trigger, I tend to be more angry than euphoric.

One thing I've found about me (and could very possibly be true for others with the same condition) is that I short cycle, but I also have long-cycling depression with it. I have noticed I feel down in the dead of winter and in the spring. Perhaps you can visualize a chart with one line in a wavy, almost methodical motion, and then you see another scribble that looks almost like an electrical bolt, very sharply pointed up and down across the wavy line. Where the two intersect, you can see the short cycling along with the condition of long-cycling depression.

Let's assume, for instance, that my business is very stressful in the spring. The promise of spring brings people out of their winter hibernation in South Dakota. They get to thinking about what they can do to increase business now that people are out and about again.

All of a sudden, after pretty much of an even level of winter work, projects come roaring in to our business. I smile and ask them when they need the work done. They reply, "Two weeks ago," or "I should have brought it in a month ago." How can you handle that situation without becoming stressed?

Additionally, I'm cycling in the spring. Spring is a kind of a low point for me. I start to get some anxiety, which means I'm burning up my medication, and I can become more depressed. On the chart you visualized, that's where the two types of lines intersect, and that's a double whammy. So when business is the most stressful, I'm almost incapable of handling the workload.

During that time, I can become more depressed—even hopeless. My self-talk is, "I'm never going to get this work done. My business is going to have to close. My wife is going to leave me." You would not believe how well I do at coming up with worst-case scenarios. If this is what goes on with me, it could also be going on with you or your loved one.

When I was single, I had most of my relationship changes in the spring. I could have a seemingly very good relationship (although who has a very good relationship with someone with my condition?), and all of a sudden I would just wake up one morning and say, "Hey, I don't want to see this person anymore."

Or I would have an episode in October. I would go through a bout of depression, usually after another rush of business orders. Like spring, fall was busy for me because people stocked up before winter set in. Since depression was already present, the added anxiety made fall really difficult on me and on those who worked and lived with me.

Try charting your moods or what is going on at certain times of the year. If you bring this information to your psychologist or your medical consultant, you may discover an adjustment or change in medication is in order.

I really don't like changing medication. As of this writing, I've lived forty years of my life with some form of cycling depression or ADHD.

I am familiar and comfortable with it. I am long cycling along with short cycling, and my short-cycle episodes can be quite intense, depending on the time of year. I've learned how to compensate for those changes.

[SK]

For Keith, the mood changes have definitely been advantageous in some ways and disadvantageous in others. He owns an intermittently successful business. However, in retrospect, he sees that he has taken on too much work himself. He's also made some business decisions that hurt him financially. He's had difficulty finding balance between his personal and professional lives. It is very difficult to find happiness in both areas of his life because there are not enough hours in the day.

Keith mentions he has down times in the spring and fall. Seasonal affective disorder (SAD) is a component of bipolar disorder and often accompanies it.

Parents of children diagnosed with mood disorders should understand how seasonal components can contribute to mood cycling. School starts in the fall and ends in the spring. The stress generated from these changes can contribute to mood swings in children and teenagers who are afflicted with mood disorders.

Whether you have the mood disorder or your loved one does, understanding that other things, like SAD, often accompany the disorder can help take some of the mystery out of why you can have so many normal days, only to be blindsided by an unexpected period of withdrawal or negativity.

Be observant. Make note if you see repetitive cycles after certain events or triggers. Work with your health care professional to find what works best in managing the mood disorder. Each patient is different and deserves as much attention to detail as it takes to help him or her live a better life.

[KC]

Obsessive/Compulsive Behavior

Dealing with obsessive/compulsive behavior has been a challenge throughout my life. The best way to explain it is like a strange form of anxiety. If I didn't pursue the behavior, I felt like something was missing or something would not be right.

My earliest recollection of obsessive/compulsive behavior was when I was five. I had a game called Cootie. There were little plastic bugs and you rolled the dice. The number determined what bug body part you received to build your Cootie. My mother told me I literally put the game away every time the exact way it had come in the box on day one—red body first, then the pink, etc. It drove me crazy if the pieces were not put away the way they came from the factory. I also recall taking the game to kindergarten. All the parts ended up in a pile at the end of playtime. I barely made it through the rest of the day.

As I grew older, the obsessive/compulsive behavior manifested in my having an interest in a hobby or subject. For instance, I became interested in astronomy. I knew all of the constellations and planets, the distance each planet was from the sun, and the makeup of the atmosphere of each planet. I even calculated the time it would take to reach each planet at the then-current speed rockets could get there—well, the projected speed. I was seven years old, and America hadn't even put a man in space at that time. My teachers were quite confused by my mathematical genius in all of this—especially since I was having a difficult time doing second-grade math assignments.

There are similar stories in my adult life. I became interested in trap shooting. The consequences seemed like life or death to me if I didn't practice. I would go out and shoot maybe two hundred rounds in the course of an hour.

Another time I bowled twelve games straight through without a break. I wasn't perfecting myself. Instead, it was like a hunger that could never be satisfied.

This may sound good to some people, and I did master a number of hobbies and work-related duties. But it's important you understand that I didn't get any internal peace from my obsessions/compulsions.

I felt no sense of accomplishment, just more drive to do what I was obsessed with. The consequences? I failed to really learn how to live a normal, balanced life. A normal life didn't fit in with my obsessions.

Looking back (and turning black and white into gray), I began to see that I could control the anxiety that was related to obsessive thoughts and compulsive behaviors. I don't have to feed the obsessions. Stop feeding the obsession, and the anxiety will pass. Spending too much time with the obsessive thoughts and compulsive behaviors also cheated me out of a balance in my work and life. It takes practice and discipline, but I truly believe my life is much more in control now.

[SK]

Anxiety and Obsessive-Compulsive Disorder

Anxiety is a part of almost every mood disorder that exists. Anxiety can be mild, like being afraid of the dark or feeling anxious about public speaking. It can also be extremely severe, such as being afraid of leaving your house or being fearful of driving. It can become so severe that it completely takes over your life. Often anxiety is the prevalent factor in obsessive-compulsive disorder. The patient becomes anxious, feeling that if a certain action is not taken, then something bad will happen. For example, a person may feel that he must wash his hands ten times or he will get sick. Someone else may feel that she has to touch each item she buys at the grocery store three times or she will get poisoned.

Imagine the time wasted in performing these rituals. Obsessive-compulsive disorder generally becomes worse if not treated.

The Saga of Chuckles the Hamster

My discussion of obsessive-compulsive disorder would not be complete without a mention of the saga of Chuckles. Chuckles was my son's hamster. Michael *loved* Chuckles. He loved Chuckles very much. In fact, Michael became obsessed with Chuckles to the point that Michael watched Chuckles night and day. Never was there a hamster more nurtured and cared for.

Michael read everything he could get his hands on about hamsters, learning about their needs for food, water, exercise, and hibernation. Included in his reading was an article that said many hamsters hibernate so deeply that people often bury them, believing they are dead. The article said that it was *very important* to make sure your hamster was dead and not in a deep state of hibernation before burying it.

Chuckles had to have exactly the right amount of water and food. He had to have exactly thirty minutes of exercise in his exercise ball twice a day (no more, no less). Of course, Chuckles had a very fancy exercise wheel in his cage, which he used at night. And, even more importantly, Chuckles' cage was kept in Michael's room where it could be watched carefully at all times.

With the tremendous amount of attention and work Chuckles received from Michael, all was very well—until one fateful evening. Unfortunately, Chuckles had a wire cage and we had a cat.

On this particular evening, I was lying in bed reading, when I suddenly heard a strange sound. I didn't know hamsters could make sounds, but I learned they definitely can. The cat had Chuckles. The cat had opened the wire cage, taken Chuckles in his mouth, and moved to the bottom of the steps, at which point I heard Chuckles' rather loud plea for help. The cat was rolling Chuckles around on the carpet.

When I saw what was going on, I called for help and the cat raced back up the steps with Chuckles in his mouth. Michael followed, completely hysterical.

Chuckles must have broken free, because the cat chased Chuckles under the bed upstairs and was in the process of scaring him to death when we were able to grab the cat. A very dazed and frightened-looking Chuckles emerged from under the bed.

Michael was totally out of sorts by then. No amount of comforting was going to help. We fixed Chuck (by now Chuckles didn't seem an appropriate name) a very comfortable bed and he seemed okay for the night (at least he was still alive).

The next morning, Michael refused to go to school because no one could watch Chuck like he could. Although I assured him I would keep Chuck right by me and keep an eye on him all day, all Michael could say was, "You will let him *die!*"

I finally convinced Michael that Chuck(les) would be okay, that I was not a hamster killer, and that he could call me at lunchtime. He reluctantly went to school.

Over the course of the day, Chuck got more lethargic. I prayed he would hold on until Michael returned from school. God forbid that Chuck should die on my watch! I called vets in town, but no one took care of hamsters. I found the only vet who treated hamsters was in Studio City, CA, which was about forty miles away. The vet worked in an animal hospital that treated all animals from the movies, including horses, elephants, and other very elite pets and animals. They agreed to take Chuck and I waited anxiously for Michael to get home from school.

When Michael arrived home from school, he took one look at Chuck and said, "Mom, we have to get Chuck to a vet *now!*"

I said that there were no vets in the area who treated hamsters, and the closest one was in Studio City. He looked at me and said, "Well, are you just gonna let him die?"

I explained that things weren't looking too good for Chuck anyway.

Michael replied, "You can't just let him die, can you?"

The hamster-killer moniker came to mind and my guilt was overwhelming. "Well, no," I said as I thought, *I am certainly* not *a hamster killer.*

And so, because I was not a hamster killer nor a child heartbreaker, I called the animal hospital in Studio City and away we went with Chuck in his cage, wrapped in a paper towel, onto the very jammed-up southern California freeway system at four o'clock rush hour.

By the time we arrived, it was 5:30 p.m. I had listened to Michael saying, "Hurry, Mom. Chuck isn't going to make it," at least five hundred times, and I was exhausted and tired of driving.

We walked into the hospital used to taking care of movie animals and put the hamster cage down in the waiting room. We were called to the back, where the examination table was large enough to hold an elephant. We were told to put the hamster on the table and the doctor would be in shortly. I hope you can get a visual of a hamster wrapped in a paper towel on an immense examination table.

When the vet entered the room, he could hardly believe what he was looking at. He gave me a very puzzled look, and I gave him a don't-you-dare-give-me-that-look look. He examined Chuck and told us it was pretty serious. Chuck had severe kidney damage, his eye was in bad shape, and so on.

Michael was hysterical.

The vet said that maybe he could save Chuck if Chuck stayed in the hospital a few days. I asked the vet if I could talk with him a few minutes, and we went out into the hall.

I told the vet that he could keep Chuck a few days, but when we returned, I wanted a hamster that looked *exactly* like Chuck, and I didn't care if it was the same hamster or not. I didn't care how much it cost, just as long as the hamster looked exactly the same. I told the vet that my son had been sick and in the hospital, and this hamster needed to *live* for everyone's sanity. I think the vet understood. At that point, I didn't really care if he got it or not.

The vet and I went back into the room, and the vet told Michael that he thought he could save Chuck, but it would take a couple of days in the hospital. The vet said Chuck needed some IV treatments. (Can you get an image of a hamster with an IV?)

The vet told us we should go home and not worry. We could call in tomorrow and he would have more news for us.

Michael and I drove home in traffic that was even worse than when we drove to Studio City earlier to Studio City in. Michael kept asking, "Do you think Chuck will be okay?" And I kept replying, "Yes, I am *sure* he will be okay," all the way home. I trusted the vet would keep his word.

At that time, I was the medical staff secretary of a hospital and had a medical staff meeting that evening at six thirty. Of course, I was an hour late.

When I arrived, the twenty-five doctors asked, "Where were you?"

I replied, "You don't want to know, trust me!" As the evening evolved, I finally told told them. They thought it was hilarious. I just glared at them all. They even asked why I hadn't brought Chuck to our hospital. I didn't think that was very funny.

The next day I called the Studio City hospital to check up on Chuck. The receptionist asked, "Do you mean Chuck the dog?"

I said, "No, not Chuck the dog."

Then she said, "Oh, you must mean Chuck the horse."

I replied, "No, not Chuck the horse."

"Well, who are you calling about?" she asked.

I felt very insecure about that question, knowing she didn't remember either me or my animal. I mean, how many hamsters did they have there? I finally answered rather quietly, "I'm calling about Chuck the *hamster.*"

Then she said, "Oh, you mean Chuck the *hamster!*" Then she laughed and said he was doing very well and getting IV steroids and had perked up quite a bit. Well, I began seeing dollar signs and asked when Chuck could come home. She told me, "Tomorrow."

The next morning I called again to see if Chuck was ready to come home. Again we went through the "which Chuck was I calling about" routine. Again I told her I was calling about Chuck the hamster. And again she said, "Oh, yes, he's doing just fine."

So, after two days of miraculous IV steroid treatments, Chuckles (now back to his full name) was ready to come home. Michael and I went to pick him up. He looked very healthy and perky, and had put on a lot of weight (steroids?). It cost me $125 (for a *hamster*, mind you), but it was worth every cent.

I never found out if it was really Chuckles for sure, but I wanted to believe it was, and he did have that little white spot on his ear, just like Chuckles did. That was the first thing Michael checked out.

Chuckles lived another three years, which is quite a long time for a hamster. I always thought it may have been the steroids, or maybe it was just the great care.

I don't think I could have handled the thought of paying $125 for a new hamster, but I always figured I had to give the vet plenty of credit for the white spot on the ear. That, in itself, was probably worth the money.

Life with Chuckles was pretty uneventful for the next three years. Of course, he got a new plastic enclosed cage.

Then, one summer morning, I heard a bloodcurdling scream from upstairs. I thought Michael had had some horrible accident, and I rushed up the stairs.

He stood in front of Chuckle's cage, sobbing. Chuckles the hamster was lying dead on his exercise wheel. It appeared to me he had been dead for some time, as he was stiff on his back on the bottom part of the wheel.

Michael looked up at me and, with pleading eyes, said, "Mom, do you think he's hibernating?"

I said, "No, Michael, I sure don't think that he is."

Then Michael said, "But the book says that they hibernate and you have to be very careful …"

I said, "Michael, I think he's pretty dead."

So Michael placed Chuckles in a shoe box and wrote a eulogy on the top lid that said, "Chuckles, you are the best pet I ever had. I will miss you forever and ever." Then he gave Chuckles a proper funeral and burial. And then I knew Chuckles was well worth everything we had invested in him.

Later, Michael got another hamster named Giggles, but it just couldn't come close to replacing Chuckles. Maybe nothing ever could.

As far as obsessive-compulsive disorder goes, my rule of thumb has always been not to treat it unless it interferes with your activities of daily living. The saga of Chuckles the hamster came close to interfering, but in the end, Michael went to school in spite of his worries about the hamster. If Michael had not gone to school, that could have been reason to treat the disorder.

I recall the case of a child who was unable to urinate if a toilet seat was a certain color. Of course, that was the color of the toilet seats at the child's school. Did that interfere with her daily living? Most definitely. Mom had to pick the child up and take her home every time she had to go to the bathroom.

All of us have some compulsive behaviors. The question is, do they interfere with life? It is up to you to decide and to take appropriate actions if they do.

There are many medications to help handle the symptoms of OCD. Discuss your problems with your physician and get help if you are experiencing difficulties that are hindering your life.

Many OCD symptoms can be treated by simply understanding that the particular ritual is part of an obsession and you have a choice. You can do it or not. Sometimes awareness that you have power over the action allows you to gain control of the ritual.

Chapter Five
Depression

[KC]

Reflecting on the depressed times, I remember feelings of not wanting to get out of bed. So many times I felt that no matter what I did, it wasn't going to do any good.

I would think about how if I stayed in bed, I wouldn't have to see anyone. I could stay isolated. The need to isolate seems to be a common thing I want to do. I don't want to be around anyone—only my machines. One reason for that is I feel that as I work, I am solving my problems. I don't know if that kind of reality is a control thing or not, but it's my reality.

As I look back, I recognize I've had this need to isolate for a long time. In relationships and while living with people, I would become extremely irritable and literally push people to the edge. Then they'd just throw their hands up and say, "That's it! I don't want anything to do with you." And I would feel good. I'd sit back and say, "Well, that's good. Them sons of bitches left me again."

I only recently realized this is a pattern I've had for years—especially when I'm at a low point and need to isolate. I'm told this could be related to abandonment issues from my past, and it can be corrected with therapy. With treatment, I have found that the need to isolate myself is really more and more a control issue—creating and controlling the environment that I, without any stress, can live in.

I see two aspects to my pushing people away when I'm feeling low. First, I don't want to be bothered by anyone, and second, I don't want to bring anyone down with me. At first I didn't think it had anything to do with control, but it really does. By isolating, I not only control others around me, I also feel in control of my surroundings. I create an environment without any stress, and I can live in it.

One of my theories about bipolars is we are constantly trying to grab at people to bring them down with us. It's an unfortunate thing because most people don't want to be brought down, but are willing to come down to our level because they love us or are concerned about us. This depressing state isn't anywhere a bipolar person really wants to be either, but we're so used to it and it's become so much a part of our lives that we literally just stay down.

When you add people to your life, you bring in different thoughts, different ideas, and different feelings. If the other person does not have bipolar disorder, he or she is even more different from you. The difference can be frustrating, so you just say, "I can't take this anymore."

Other people, especially women, have always added stress for me. For example, before I was married, I only felt comfortable or at ease with women during sexual activity. Does that mean that in the past, women were nothing more than sex objects to me? In the past, yes, very much so. I literally had relationships in which I felt all the woman was good for was sex. If I let her into my world, she would disrupt things, and I'd have to consider someone else besides me. That stressed me out and I didn't want that.

It was easier for me to be isolated. The responsibility that it takes to have a relationship, coupled with my heightened sense of failure if I did not deal with my perfectionist standards, depressed me. I was used to giving 110 percent in everything I did. In a relationship, I expected to make someone happy 110 percent of the time, and there's no way to do that. It's not going to happen. Both of you are going to have your lows and your highs. Unless you both cycle at the same time, you may be in an up mood while the other person could be in a down mood. And from what I've seen in relationships bipolars have, that is what it seems like—the bipolar person drags the other person down.

Misconception

There's a misconception that the bipolar person really wants to be isolated—to be left alone. The reality is the bipolar person, specifically me, wants an environment that is predictable, that feels safe, and that doesn't require the responsibility of motivating and dealing with other people. Generally, relationships do not offer that type of stability and predictability. This triggers anxiety and mood swings in the bipolar person.

[SK]

I have often seen people like Keith in my practice. It's very difficult for them to accept the unpredictable nature of relationships. There are no guarantees in love, and people with control issues find this difficult to accept. They are used to going to work, working a certain number of hours, and getting a paycheck. They save up a certain amount of money and buy a house. They do their homework, study hard and get a good grade. That is how life is. But in relationships, it doesn't work that way and that's difficult to accept. A person can vow unending love one day and walk out the next, or even threaten to end the relationship one day and rekindle the flame the next. *There are no guarantees!* This is extremely difficult for a person who is used to being in charge of his or her life.

Many people who are unable to let go of this need to control find it easier not to be in a relationship at all because it is too difficult for them to trust the uncertainty.

[KC]

Dark Thoughts

Before I leave the topic of depression and isolation, I want to share my experience with dark thoughts. I warn you that this section can be disturbing to read, but this book is about giving you the perspective of a bipolar person working his way from the dark times into the light.

I've spent years searching for windows of normal that I never had. I've lived my life in a little box for no reason I knew. I became accustomed to it and wore my constricted bipolar states like a tight corset. After years of working toward getting better, I now know it's possible.

I've learned to breathe the air without life support, and you or your loved one can too. When you read this section about my dark thoughts, you'll know that if I can get better, your situation is not hopeless. And that, after all, is the whole purpose for writing this book.

I don't know if it's in every bipolar personality to have dark thoughts or other conditions in which dark thoughts are involved, but I feel that dark thoughts can actually become a ritual or a habit.

The medical world may disagree with me on this because they think a person can take more antidepressants or more mood stabilizers to make the dark thoughts go away. My opinion is that you can drug yourself into oblivion, but what has become ritualized or a practiced habit is hard to break—even with medication.

The one thing I did notice is that when I took mood stabilizers and antianxiety medicines, the dark thoughts still came, but I was able to realize they were dark thoughts, and I made a good attempt at shutting them off. The sad thing about dark thoughts is they become such a ritual that they come back to us when we get stressed.

Unfortunately, what usually happens is the dark thoughts get spewed onto the people you love the most—your family, close friends, significant other, and in general the people you think are there in your corner, pulling for you.

The real harm in dark thoughts comes because the thoughts do multiple levels of damage. Your dark thoughts can scare people. I notice I like the shock value they produce. That's one level.

Then there's the isolation factor. When I want to be alone, I like spewing dark thoughts to get the isolation mode in gear. I've been in relationships and been told, "You're the most unhappy person in the world." Before I got treatment, I thought, *Oh yeah? I'm in the real world. So what's wrong with you?* And in many ways I did think I was in the real world. But spewing out dark thoughts of death and destruction is really nonproductive.

As I started to deal with my dark thoughts, I realized they were going to occur. Working with treatment and medication can really help in the sense that you learn you do not have to live with dark thoughts twenty-four hours a day, as I did. Before medication, a typical day for me was to wake up in the morning and think dark thoughts. I would go on to work through the day, and everything continued to be negative and dark thoughts.

After the mood stabilizers and antianxiety medicine, I have more control. I may start thinking dark thoughts, and may even get through thirty seconds to a minute of them before I think, "Wait a minute. Now wait just one darn minute. Quit wasting your time thinking about these things."

I know many people—my spouse, my therapist, and such—have always asked me that. "Why do you waste your time with them?" I think the answer comes from the fact that dark thoughts are useful for shock value and for spewing out. When you want to be alone, sharing the dark thoughts programs people to do just that—leave you alone.

Besides being useful for pushing people away from you, dark thoughts give you a sense of control in your life, which is something you're striving for. The only way to get control is to become isolated, a huge issue for bipolars. We don't want to deal with people when we're down, but actually, that's when we need the most help.

Medication can level out your moods, but any little trigger—stress, words someone said, and so on—can trigger the dark thoughts again.

I guess being able to recognize what triggers you helps, because then you can say to yourself, "Well, I'm not going to be bothered by this, so I'll just think of something else."

It's unfortunate for me that I've carried these dark thoughts most of my life and they are just ingrained in my psyche. The result of thinking them is I spewed them out to my mother and my wife. Much of it has been to see the shock value—to just blow everybody out of my way so I can get control.

To get out of my ritual of dark thoughts, I tried many things. The first thing I did was martial arts breathing. I can even do this when I'm driving in my car. I breathe in through my nose, breathing low, distending my abdomen, pushing the air low into my lungs, blowing it out, taking another deep breath, and finally exhaling through my mouth. At the same time, I envision the breath coming into my nostrils like a clean, fine mist, going down my windpipe, circulating through my body, and then coming out through my mouth. I keep breathing and visualizing for twenty cycles. And I notice I feel better. It seems like the oxygen is changing brain waves and patterns. But what it also does is work out that stabbing feeling in my stomach.

That helps turn my thoughts from my troubles, and I can think, "I'm going to a safe place. I'm on my grandparents' farm again." I visualize the things I remember from the farm, the smells, the sun on my face, and the smells in Grandma's kitchen. It's all there.

What's really going on is I'm breaking the pattern. You know what it's like. You're driving along, intent on getting home, when all of a sudden you remember you're supposed to pick up the dry cleaning. What did remembering that do? It broke the pattern. Or let's say you're thinking about a project. You're very engrossed in your thoughts about work when all of a sudden you remember about picking up the dry cleaning. BOOM! You broke your thought pattern.

When I'm in the depressed state, I'm extremely negative. By learning to break the pattern even slightly, I can back off the dark thoughts and realize what's going on. I can ask myself why I am depressed. I have to stop and think, and what really takes courage is to say, "Yep,

47

I am responsible for the dark thoughts, so now what am I going to do about them?" Breathing is important because it brings oxygen into your brain, and visualizing the safe place is very important because it puts you in a happier place.

Some people suggest that I think about the fact that other people have it worse than I do. Well, my reaction is, who cares?

Your main objective needs to be to get yourself out of the depressed state. The longer you stay in it, the more chance you have of hurting yourself or just plain getting lethargic and tired and then going backward.

When you start the backward slide, think things through. And try to keep your mouth shut around your spouse. I caught myself acting out the dark-thought rituals around my wife, and I stopped.

It's also important to reflect on what your triggers are. For me, I can just look at certain people and become completely infuriated. But I remind myself I am in control, and it works.

Dark thoughts are rituals that can become extremely frightening. I would often go into a fight-or-flight mode. When I say fight, I mean extreme dark thoughts like murder, murdering families—horrible, horrible thoughts, and I know they are horrible.

And that's the beauty of getting on medication. I can actually look back and say, "Hey, wait a minute." Unfortunately, the dark thoughts still have a profound mood effect on me. I have to say, "I am not going to let [whatever] bother me. I am not going to hold it in."

You see, that's another problem. Holding these negative feelings in is no good either, because all it does is create more toxic waste. Eventually that toxic waste has to be disposed of—released. Usually the way it's disposed of is by spewing it all over family members.

You can emotionally discipline yourself and say, "Okay, I'm not going to let even the sight of this person bother me any longer. I am not going to be affected by this negativity. I am going to go on with my life."

The medication is not going to cure you from being yourself. It is, however, going to help you with the physiological issues that you have to deal with, which, in turn, helps you with the psychological issues. You have to correct the behavioral problems yourself. If you want to build your biceps, you don't just all of a sudden have twenty-one-inch biceps overnight. You work on that area. And that's the way it is with changing yourself. You work on an area a little at a time, and you keep working.

[SK]

I've found that dark thoughts are experienced by a tremendously large population of bipolar and obsessive-compulsive people. These people are often terrified of the thoughts. Dark thoughts are rarely discussed openly and honestly the way Keith has defined them. I've had many patients who are extremely troubled by dark thoughts. Keith's candid discussion, although very difficult, catches the essence of the dark side of the thought processes suffered by so many patients. I hope his sharing will bring comfort to those who've experienced dark thoughts, especially regarding how those thoughts affect people with bipolar disorder.

Chapter Six
Structure

[SK]

People with bipolar disorder need structure. In today's hectic world, structure can be difficult for them and for those around them. The more closely a daily routine can be followed, the better.

Structure means mealtimes, bedtimes, and medication times (and dosages) should be consistent, whether the patient is feeling manic, depressed, or in between.

A diet high in protein, including high-protein snacks, eaten at frequent intervals, provides optimal mood stabilization. Some people eat a small amount of protein before getting out of bed in the morning and then again every two to three hours throughout the day.

Aerobic exercise also helps to keep moods stable. It is important to note that twenty to thirty minutes of aerobic exercise every twenty-four hours is the most beneficial way to help with mood stabilization, because that amount of exercise causes the release of endorphins. Endorphins, chemically speaking, are the precursor to morphine, which is very similar to serotonin, the feel-good receptor in the brain. However, because this effect lasts for only twenty-four hours, it is important to release the endorphins every twenty-four hours. Thus, a twenty- to thirty-minute exercise program every twenty-four hours is the ideal for improving and stabilizing moods.

Some have suggested that supplements such as Omega 3 fish oil taken during the day may help to keep moods under control. GABA is an amino acid that often helps to calm people. However, it is important to check with your doctor before introducing any supplements to your regimen.

If you live in a climate with long winters, sun lamps can help tremendously with seasonal affective depression episodes. You can purchase sun lamps from many places, including the Internet.

A consistent sleep time (and waking time) is also important, although very difficult to achieve for most bipolar patients. Relaxation, guided imagery, and hypnosis CDs can all be helpful in overcoming sleep problems.

Children Need Structure Too

Structure is not only important to adult patients, it is necessary for children diagnosed with bipolar disorder, ADHD, Tourette syndrome, OCD, and/or dyslexia. The more closely you can follow a consistent daily routine, the better for you and your child.

Make sure you serve meals at the same time every day. Many parents claim that a breakfast high in protein, and morning snacks of cheese, nuts, or any other type of protein, help control moods. Continue to give these high-protein snacks every few hours through the day.

You'll also want to create and maintain an environment that is structured, relaxed, and quiet for your child. A consistent time for doing homework is best. It's also wise to allow the child to choose the time he or she thinks is best for study. Once the time is selected, you can more easily enforce the time because the child has had some control in establishing the process.

One thing we cannot control in terms of structure is the outside temperature. Children with bipolar disorder and ADHD have a tendency to become extremely hot when it's *not* hot outside. They go out without coats; they go barefoot in the winter. They don't get sick, they just run hot. I mention this because you may not be aware that many other parents deal with this problem too.

Another thing you may think is unusual, but really isn't, is children with mood disorders have a sensitivity to clothing. Even if you cut the labels out, the child may complain the clothes "itch." The feeling is probably the result of tactile hypersensitivity. The solution is fabric softener. Sweatpants and sweatshirts or t-shirts often help too. Most children outgrow this by the time they are in junior or senior high school (or maybe vanity overrules comfort).

The last thing I want to discuss under the topic of structure is discipline. I have three guidelines when it comes to disciplining a child with any mood disorder. First, choose your battles. Second, be consistent. Third, remember that negative reinforcement generally does not work with these children. Therefore, learn all you can about positive reinforcement.

Choose Your Battles

You will have many issues to deal with, so it's smart to select which battles you want to fight. Is it *really* that important your child eat *all* that spinach? Does the child's bedroom *really* need to be cleaned *every* week? Maybe your child must be dressed and ready to go to school at 8:15 a.m. every day. Fight that battle. Maybe your son should stop biting his sister. Fight that battle. You're the parent, and your priorities are different from some other parents', so you need to decide which battles are important and which aren't.

When you're determining your priorities, develop your discipline plan. Decide which behaviors you want to change first. That's what priorities are all about. If you target too many at one time, you will overwhelm your child and frustrate yourself. How many behaviors are too many? That depends on the age and maturity level of your child. Usually three to five behaviors are plenty. Again, depending on the age and maturity level of your child, you may even allow your child to help you determine which behaviors to work on changing.

Once you've selected the behaviors, it is important to make a chart. These children are generally very visual. They are unable to remember to do things unless they *see* them. List the targeted behavior and the days of the week. Get some stars or stickers. When your child completes the targeted behavior, place a star or sticker in the corresponding box so the child can see the accomplishment.

When a certain number of stars or stickers are earned and placed on the chart, reward the child. The reward does not have to be costly. It can be a picnic with Mom and Dad in a local park, for example. It must be something the child will enjoy. Some parents have grab bags of inexpensive toys. Others offer quarters or even a dollar.

When you write the targeted behavior, it's very important that you are specific. To write "Brush your teeth morning and night" is fine—specific. To write "Clean your room" is too vague because the child doesn't know what that means exactly.

Once the child has mastered a behavior, add another to the chart. Let the child know the more behaviors the child masters, the more rewards the child can earn. I often tell parents that positive reinforcement is a nice, clinical word for bribery, but it works and we *always* refer to it as positive reinforcement because that term sounds so much better.

Be Consistent

Both parents must be consistent with the child. These children are master manipulators and will try everything to break you down. Of course you love your child. That's exactly why both of you are going to work together on being consistent. You want your child to have a chance at life and all the possibilities it holds for them with their intelligence and creativity. Stay united and your child wins. Become inconsistent and you risk a lot.

Negative Reinforcement Doesn't Work

This is a system of *positive reinforcement*, and it works for all children, no matter what their age. Negative reinforcement doesn't work because children with mood disorders don't understand why you took something away from them. They don't learn anything positive; they only become extremely angry and uncooperative.

It's easy to turn a negative reinforcement into a positive one. For example, when the child is old enough to drive, keep the car keys rather than giving a set to the child. The car belongs to *you*. If the child has the car keys and misbehaves, then you have to be the bad guy and take the keys away. When you flip that dynamic around and you have the keys, then if the child behaves, you can be the benevolent parent who allows the child to borrow the keys. Same outcome, but a different mechanism of parental control. If you are creative, you can change almost everything into a positive situation and your life will be much easier. I'm a parent who's done this, and I know that it works.

Structure is one of the least expensive ways you can help your loved one. Structure may also be one of the best ways to help yourself. Who knows? You may even create a little reward system for you as you monitor your own efforts to understand and support your loved one.

CHAPTER SEVEN
MANIC STATES

[KC]

This chapter starts with a reflection about the feeling (emotional and physical) of a manic state that was inadvertently induced by a medication change. I include this chapter to help you. If you have been on medication and all of a sudden you feel triggers like I describe below, call someone. If you are alone, understand what is going on with you and try to suppress things.

I was doing quite well with the cycling. I was on BuSpar, Lamictal, and Wellbutrin.

I had been having some irritability problems, and the psychiatrist thought that possibly the antianxiety medication was counteracting the mood stabilizer. Thus, my medications were modified.

Within eight hours, I was heading into a full-blown manic state.

By now you know I own a business. I was working on projects that were not going well. I recall feeling that everyone I worked with was totally inferior. I mean, I even quipped, "I wish I could drill a hole in these people's heads and pour my brain into them." I was becoming zero tolerant.

Then I began to have a heightened sensory perception. I was at a luncheon meeting, and people eating across the room sounded like they were chewing directly into my ear through a bullhorn. I became extremely irritable and agitated. I wasn't recognizing what was happening to me was that I was heading into a full manic state.

For me, a full manic state is not a euphoric place. It is a place laden with self-hate, self-pity, self-fear, and often self-mutilation.

Because I was under the care and working under the direction of a health care professional and being treated with medication, I just assumed this feeling would pass. Well, it didn't pass. It got worse.

My evening was relaxing and nondescript. After supper, I had approximately two ounces of alcohol in a mixed drink, and I settled down to watch a movie at home. After the movie, I got up and prepared for bed. I began reading a book.

All of a sudden, I felt like snakes were crawling inside my stomach. A feeling of complete dread began to arise, as well as old feelings of abandonment and self-hatred.

Prior to that, as I mentioned, I had been irritable at work. I even did some self-mutilating. The self-mutilation consisted of slapping myself and hitting myself in the face, which was rather unique, but it didn't leave any marks.

Someone asked me once if the self-mutilation helped me feel relief or anything. For me, self-mutilation in my manic state is a punishment. I say to myself, "Why did you get here? You deserve to be punished." And I become an outside person doing the punishing.

[SK]

Keith's form of self-mutilation and his reasoning for it are somewhat unusual compared to what most self-mutilating patients report. When asked why they cut themselves or self-mutilate, they usually state that they either want to "feel something—anything," or they want to "shut off or divert the emotional pain" they are feeling. By feeling physical pain, they can shut off their emotional pain for a while. Keith's explanation of self-punishment, while not unheard of, is certainly not a common explanation.

Cutting, burning, or other self-injurious behaviors are becoming more and more common, especially in young women. One of the most recently identified self-injurious behaviors is using repetitive motions with erasers to cause burns on the skin. These raised, red areas, which sometimes split the skin, are extremely prone to infection and hurt more than anticipated by the patient.

For some, self-injurious behavior is a way to divert the emotional pain and relieve anxiety and stress. For others who feel numb, it is a way to feel something and prove they are alive. The patients are aware that the behavior makes no sense. However, they are helpless to stop it.

Numerous Web sites discuss self-injurious behavior, and while these sites can be helpful for professionals, they often trigger afflicted persons to injure themselves. Self-injurious behavior was once shrouded in secrecy and shame. However, that has changed as more Web sites talk openly about it. Sadly, some teens think self-mutilation is trendy and do it to fit in with peers, which is a cause for great concern and parents should be aware of this.

However, bipolar patients remain the most likely to participate in self-injurious behavior. Because of the extreme intensity of emotions felt by bipolars, self-injurious behavior is very popular among them. When the patient is in a manic state, self-injuring can turn off emotional chaos and divert it to physical pain. When in a depressed phase, self-injurious behavior can allow the patient to feel something besides numbness.

More self-mutilators are female than male. Many also have eating disorders or suicidal tendencies, although self-mutilation in itself is not considered a suicide attempt.

Perhaps the most common form of self-injury is cutting. It is said to relieve stress, and it becomes a part of the daily routine. Cutters claim to get a rush from it that allows them to get through the day. This rush is most likely related to a release of adrenaline.

Other methods of self-injurious behavior are more subtle and can include banging one's head, hitting oneself, driving unusually fast, or even becoming angry with little provocation. All of these behaviors are adrenaline-seeking and often result in outcomes similar to cutting.

It is extremely difficult for family members to understand why a person would want to inflict pain on him or herself. After all, we are creatures who generally avoid pain and dangerous situations. It is essential to understand this behavior is common in bipolar patients (as well as in some others) because it:

1. Gives the patient a little adrenaline rush, which patients report helps them to get through the day.

2. Relieves emotional stress or pain by forcing the patient to concentrate on on a physical sensation.

3. Allows them to feel something if they have been numb.

Self-mutilation can occur in anyone because, sadly, some socially isolated kids participate in this behavior just to get attention and/or to belong to a group.

[KC]

The actual manic state was terrible. I felt extremely agitated and fearful. I woke my wife and began to carry on. Over and over again I went on about my fears of abandonment, my fears other men were better than me, my wanting to be them. I kept going until I began a frenzy of hitting my face.

It was intense and completely irrational. It was almost a euphoric feeling, if self-hatred can be euphoric. I got up and walked around several times. I screamed. I paced the floor.

[SK]

Again, Keith returned to his comfortable "friend"—self-medication with alcohol—which had been his comfort zone for so many years. This is a natural tendency for a bipolar who is newly diagnosed, properly medicated, and has had to cope for so many years without proper medical treatment.

[KC]

After you come down from one of these manic states, there is a certain form of remorse and panic you need to address.

The first remorse is the turmoil you put your family through. I look back and see that I did this all the time—for more than twenty years. It's almost like living in a form of purgatory. You do not understand what is going on with you, and you need help.

I can still feel my skin crawl. I can still feel my brain exploding in my head. I can still feel the almost-need to take a blade and stick it into my churning lower abdomen. That was scary; that was definitely scary.

Prior to treatment, there were many things I would have done to seek an adrenaline rush. Some of these things (maybe family members can relate to these) included drinking binges or driving my car as fast as it would allow me to go and taking curves as fast as I could. What I was doing was dumping adrenaline, basically dousing a fire with gasoline.

Family Involvement

When you find yourself in a manic state, or you begin to notice the triggers, try to not make any major decisions. Any decisions you make will be based more on emotion than fact.

One of the suggestions I made to my family is that when they first notice the extreme irritability or negativity, they can make me aware of it by asking questions like, "Has the medication changed?" or "Has there been something different?"

You almost have to set up an action plan with your family, because if you go completely over the edge, like I did, you will either end up in an emergency room or staying overnight, even up to a week, at a psychiatric facility.

If you feel you want to do or are beginning to do self-harm, you have to find help immediately because you are too close to the edge. You cannot push yourself to the point of no return. There is no going back.

And watch your decisions. Just say to yourself, "I am not going to make any decisions here." That statement includes, "I am not going to make a decision to hurt myself."

You have to take into consideration your immediate family. If you are living alone and do not have any immediate family around you, take yourself into consideration. You may live alone, but you do not live in a vacuum. You have people who love you and worry about you. You have people who rely on you to be there—perhaps an employer, perhaps a neighbor, perhaps a friend. And if you have a pet, you really need to take care of yourself so your beloved pet has a home. If you harm yourself and have to go to a psychiatric ward for a few days or even a week, who would even know that your dog or cat was left alone?

If you won't take care of yourself for you, think of those around you. Just because you live alone doesn't mean you *are* alone.

I know this is difficult, especially in a manic state. Until I began to see things turn from black and white into gray, I didn't care if I was dead or alive. I was not going to pull a trigger, but if I had seen a bus coming, I might have just stood there without getting out of the way.

Family members have the impossible burden of reasoning with the manic person, a task that is difficult at best and impossible at worst.

Family members: no matter what, don't let the bipolar person leave you. That person is either going out to seek tremendous amounts of alcohol or other drugs to pull himself down, or he is going after an adrenaline rush. Either choice can kill him. Whether the adrenaline comes from promiscuous sexual activity or other dangerous acts, the bipolar person is trying to feel like he does not or will not care about the very thing he cares about, which is seeking that "window." He is searching for calm, not adrenaline. It's a kind of strange thing. The best way to describe it is that you're scared, and you bring in some other thing that's going to scare you worse so you can forget about what you're normally scared of.

The main thing to understand is how literally incoherent you are at this point. Unfortunately, in my life as an adult and as a businessman, I would say I have spent three-quarters of my time either manic or depressed. Rarely was I in the middle.

It's scary when things are out of control. When I first started thinking I was coming back to the middle, I'd say to myself, "Hey, I'm back and I'm working hard! I'm getting things done again." Was I? No, I was not. I was constantly bombarded with racing thoughts and anger. I got nothing done. I maybe had some insight, but that was all.

[SK]

I think people who are in a manic state may have a false sense of achievement. They feel they are getting a lot done. This may be true, but then they cycle down, and much of what was gained is often lost. It therefore is often a vicious cycle of getting a great deal done, making frequent mistakes, correcting the mistakes, and then crashing down into a place where little is accomplished over a period of time. One is always seeking to find that mode of being able to get things accomplished again.

[KC]

When I get on an even keel, I try to stay focused. One thing I used to do is have manic states three times a week. Those were the times when I grew my business the fastest. That's all fine and dandy, but I do not feel that it's healthy, and it is definitely not healthy for a family setting.

If you can eliminate the anxiety, I think that's a start to keeping oneself on that even path. It is strange, however, that at first the drugs put me on an even path, and I did not want to stay there. It seemed like I became more depressed as time went on.

Now I often wonder if finding healthy activities, such as exercise or possibly getting back into karate again, could help me achieve a positive form of the manic state.

For me, however, the manic state is not euphoric. It is not a good thing. It is filled with panic, fear, despair, and hopelessness. As I search for the even keel, I feel that my body, as it tries to get out of the depressed mode, begins to climb and then almost climbs over the edge in its effort to get to the normal side.

While preparing to write this section and progressively studying the after-manic state, it became apparent to me how I cycle. I understand weekly cycling now—by the end of the week, my creativity and my ability to handle irritation begin to subside.

As I reflect over the years, I see I would cycle twice a week. One major catastrophe on Wednesday would usually carry me to the weekend. The other disaster came when I cycled on the weekends. After winding down, I'd get to the point where I would be ready to go into a manic state again.

If you feel something like this is happening to you, just being aware of it is very helpful.

Now I'm working at staying put together. For example, I have a business networking meeting that I go to even though I find it dreadful. It used to be made up of people who offered a lot of motivation and positive input. Most of those people have left the group now. There is a new administration that is much more rigid. Sometimes I get so irritated with this meeting that I become hypersensitive. The people across the room who are chewing on their food sound like they are chewing in my ear. But now I recognize that's really my body trying to deal with a manic state.

The best way I'm finding to handle the situation is to tell myself that this is not an upbeat place anymore, but I can make changes. I can feel upbeat, I can sit back and talk in a friendly way to people, and maybe I can change the meeting around. I don't want to take full responsibility for changing it, but it's a fact that I can change the way I perceive things.

I think bipolars all see the world differently. Some view it as euphoric, almost a dreamland. Others, like me, view life as a place to kill or be killed. This can be somewhat helpful, because you can work under more pressure than the average person and your body is used to it—your body craves adrenaline.

Think about it. You are trying to progress through life, trying to find that "window of normal." If you recognize that you can change the way you perceive things, you can at least make an attempt to stay in a middle ground.

Enlightenment

I call the window of time when I can function without some of the negative symptoms *enlightenment*. In order not to lose my enlightenment, I find it helpful to sit back and try to look at both sides of an issue.

For example, in my small business, I sometimes deal with too many phone calls and too much problem solving. At least that's the way I feel about it. Recently I was trying to get through to certain people. In today's world, we communicate mostly through voice mail and e-mail. Many times, I find I grow impatient with this.

As an effect of my increasing impatience, I was transitioning from an enlightened state and heading toward a manic state. I was mindful of that. I was trying to get through to a certain salesperson, and I got voicemail. Right away, my normal response to this trigger was, "Oh boy, here we go again. Can never get a hold of anybody. What a messed up world!" Then I said, "Hey, wait a minute. It's the same way for other people trying to get a hold of me!" And that's true when I'm in a bad mood and I won't speak to people.

I came to the realization that I am no different from anyone else, and I can't change society or people. It's easy for people to say how enlightened I am, even though I am a person with bipolar issues. I'm venturing out of my little shell, and it's helpful to realize there are going to be irritations. I try to look at the other side of the coin, to put myself in the comparison. How are people reacting to me?

It also helps to think of good things when the hopeless, negative thoughts come to mind. Again, you can go to your safe place, use positive affirmation, and so on. I've been told you cannot hold both a positive and a negative thought in your mind at the same time.

I recognize we can't sit around all the time saying, "Everything is good. Everything is positive." But the idea is to *try*, and I do mean try, because it is not going to be easy putting positive thoughts in your mind when you're used to being negative.

It Takes Work
One thing that's imperative to understand is a bipolar can wish and hope all he wants to get better, but it takes work. The medication can get you so far. The rest takes training inside yourself. You have to learn to react to your environment in a different way. You have to break the habitual behavior. You have to learn to identify your triggers, to know when these triggers are hitting you, and train yourself to stop the triggers. How you react is almost a ritual, and you have to learn new rituals.

I used to think, "I'm not this and I'm not that because of my training. And I'm not this and I'm not that because I had a crappy life, my mom whacked out on me, and my dad killed himself. It's all their fault."

Yes, I have been trained to react negatively to most situations. I became programmed to expect failure more than success. As I said earlier, I expected the best, but prepared for the worst. Always preparing for the worst programmed me so that I could make the worst happen. Sound crazy? Well, it is, but it's also the truth. When you think negatively, you're going to get negative results.

It isn't so much that you create negative instances. You more or less program your life into your thinking that everything is going to be negative. I'm the first one to realize that. I'm the first one to sit back and say, "Now, wait a minute. I am assuming this is going to turn out negative, so I am looking for all the negative possible outcomes to that situation."

When you finally figure out you have a mood disorder, you think, "Well, I'm bipolar and I'm going to react this way and I'm going to have a negative state of mind." I thought that way all the time.

With training, as time goes on, you will not find yourself thinking as much about putting the positive thoughts into your mind. It will just happen. You will have trained your mind enough. NOTE: Do not drop your medication at this point. You will feel good. You will feel better. But you are far from being better completely.

Manic states can be pretty scary for both the patient and the family. Create a plan with your family before the manic state hits. That way, they know what to do to help you. If you're alone, take care of yourself so you're there for those who love and need you.

You can learn to spend more time in the middle ground, but it takes more than medication. It takes work, and you can do it. You can reprogram your negative thoughts into positive ones. You can reset your triggers before they set you off. You can train yourself, and it's worth the effort.

CHAPTER EIGHT
CHANGES

[KC]

In the last chapter, I said you cannot think a positive thought and a negative thought at the same time. As you work on reprogramming your thinking rituals, you'll find more positive thoughts taking the place of the negative. You will have trained your mind enough that negative thoughts will actually become a thing of the past.

But there's always the possibility of going back into a manic state. I think that the majority of the time, a manic state happens because we've conditioned our minds to become manic. Even though we have medication, the manic state returns.

There was a point when I couldn't think any positive thoughts, couldn't even laugh. It was interesting when people first met me. I came across as positive, but I was conditioning myself. I was acting to keep these new people mesmerized for a time. Then, as relationships grew—friendships, male/female relationships, dating, and especially marriage—the real me popped out, and sometimes what popped out could be very startling, like a scary jack-in-the-box.

People are creatures of habit, and for the most part, none of us likes change. Especially for a bipolar, change is very frightening. Most of our behavior is habitual, and even the reaction of family members is habitual. Family members can push bipolars over the edge, depress them, or react in a way that encourages them to be totally unstable. My point is that family members have to examine their own behaviors and change their habits along with the bipolar person.

Safe Place

I talked in an earlier chapter about bipolars visualizing a safe place. But know that even if you create a safe place, it won't always work. You will sometimes find a way to mess things up.

After thinking about how my manic states were somewhat controllable when I had the awareness that I could go into a manic state, I inadvertently did a bit of an experiment.

Previously I said that whatever you do, even if you become enlightened, do not give up taking your medication. One day I got busy and forgot to take my meds. No antianxiety, no Wellbutrin, no mood stabilizer. By early afternoon, I was back to my old behavior. Even though I was somewhat coherent, I became very irritable and extremely impatient.

So I say again that even if you think you can go off your meds, even though you are emotionally in control, don't try it. Don't even try weaning off of them. Even though you feel better, even though you're aware of what's going on with you, *do not stop taking your medications.* I think 60 percent of how you feel is medication and 40 percent is your attitude, your awareness, and what you do about it.

Three Phases of Medication Therapy

Once you get your medication stabilized, you can move ahead and look at your life. During my years of drug therapy and counseling, I experienced three phases.

1. *Denial that I was suffering from any form of chemical imbalance or malfunction.* You fight those ideas, and you fight the fact that you don't want to take treatment. I've been told that after they learn they have a mood

disorder, most people will not take treatment for at least six months.

2. *Fighting the medication.* Your body is rebelling against feeling good. It has felt bad for so long that it does not even know how to begin the process of returning to normal. My experience was I went through at least six months of experimentation with psychiatric medications because of how my body reacted. I finally hit a plateau while taking a mild antidepressant and a mood stabilizer. Once I got the proper combination, I did well. For me, it appears that 60 percent of my issues were caused by a chemical imbalance, leaving 40 percent of my issues being caused by my ritualized or ingrained behavior.

3. *Guilt rounds out the three phases.* All of a sudden, you start to feel better. As you review your life, you find a tremendous amount of guilt. It may begin to push you into manic states from time to time because you cannot function under the burden of guilt. Guilt is anxiety. Guilt is stress.

[SK]

Many bipolars are reluctant to take medication because they have become used to dealing with their unstable moods. They enjoy the energy associated with the manic states and are often willing to suffer the lows in order to keep the highs. It is therefore often difficult to convince them of the need for medication. Many feel dull on medication. Many are diagnosed later in life and have found other ways to cope with their ups and downs. It is a difficult and personal decision to determine whether to live on an even keel or to continue on a roller-coaster ride, but it is a decision that every diagnosed bipolar must make.

As Keith mentions above, many treated bipolars experience tremendous guilt. Guilt is extremely destructive. It is an emotion that eats away at the psyche and destroys it a day at a time. It is very important for healing bipolars to address, explore, and deal with their feelings of guilt. Sometimes this means making amends or peace with people who have been hurt by prior behavior. Eliminating guilt is an essential part of treatment and healing that is often overlooked and can cause years of future problems.

[KC]

Guilt can pass as you mentally exercise. You know your past life is littered with broken relationships, hurt feelings, and many times, with hurting yourself—emotionally or even physically. You or loved ones probably still carry scars internally.

A minister told me once that your mind keeps playing back the times when you hurt somebody. I suppose the same is true for when you hurt yourself. Then the minister said, "It's God's way of keeping you from doing it again, reminding you that this type of behavior is not acceptable."

When you get moving again, you'll see it and understand how guilt can pass.

After you become aware of what's going on with you, or when you are actually getting better, you may still experience a need for isolation.

But rather than becoming isolated because you're depressed, as I talked about in an earlier chapter, you need isolation because of something that happened. You may see that you have wronged people in the past. Or maybe you behaved inappropriately. Either way, you may try to put yourself in a self-imposed exile. You may feel you have done so many wrong things that you cannot, no matter how much your family or friends care about you, live with it.

After medication, such thoughts are more controllable, but there's still a guilt thing, like you don't deserve to be with these people. You also don't want to harm them anymore. If you make yourself aware of this, it's easier to deal with, although the thoughts will still cross your mind.

The bottom line is that isolation will remain part of your psyche. But remember, it is mostly a learned behavior. The main thing is to remember that you cannot let guilt consume you. You have to fight it. You have to say to yourself, "No, I am not going to allow myself to punish myself in this way."

Self-punishment, self-mutilation, and harmful behaviors can all create a situation where you feel people just can't take you anymore. Before I knew what was wrong with me and began treatment, I just didn't care. My mantra was "Accept me for who I am." I didn't feel any form of acceptance. My thought pattern was, "Hey people, this is the way it is—take it or leave it." And unfortunately it became a cycle, just like my moods.

[SK]

It is extremely confusing for the people around bipolars to understand the behaviors associated with the disorder. Often family and friends search for reasons for self-mutilation or rages. It is difficult to understand that these behaviors may have nothing to do with anything external, but are simply a part of the internal thought processes and mood cycles of the bipolar. Perhaps more a defense mechanism or manifestation of frustration, at times self-mutilating behavior can be a form of self-punishment for causing too much pain to others or frustration for having done so.

However, in my experience, most self-mutilation is performed because a patient either wants to feel something or wants to divert intense emotional feelings.

Self-mutilating behavior, although relatively common, is just beginning to be addressed in books, and especially in association with bipolar illness. I believe it is a huge red flag for bipolar illness for the above reasons. Although not all bipolars self-mutilate, a percentage of them do, and professionals should be aware that it can be a part of the clinical spectrum of the disorder.

[KC]

The people closest to you are still drawn to you by their caring and your ability. As my wife put it, "The good times were very good and the bad times were very bad." Most people remember the good times over the bad, which is good for those of us who help create the bad times. Even though most people remember the good, our guilt may overcome us, and that's what sends us into self-imposed exile—another learned behavior.

Control

Let's say I have gotten into something that I don't have total control of, and it makes me feel panic. My self-talk is, "How could you be so stupid as to agree to this?" It's like always being on automatic pilot and then having a feeling of worthlessness. When you're on automatic pilot, you don't have control.

But you can take back control—control of your mind and control of the fact that the first thing you have to work on is spewing negativity all over people.

I'm not saying you should push your anger down. I'm saying you can control and direct your energy to the positive side, or you can file that energy in the negative filing cabinet. People may tell you to just let the negative go and forget all about it, but that's not necessarily what happens. Sometimes you need negative energy.

Let's assume the same opportunity came up and I had a negative experience, as was the case in a business dealing I had. Well, some might say, forget about it. Life is positive. I don't think this will happen again. I filed the negative away and put the stops in.

The point is that not all negative experiences are bad or need to be forgotten. They can be filed away and kept for future reference. The goal is to reframe them as much as possible, changing the habit from negative thinking to positive thinking.

As you're working on control issues, there may come a time when you start feeling hate. It isn't hate for another person. It's self-hate, which is probably one of the most damaging thought processes ever. When you self-hate, you completely lose control. Think about it. When you direct hate at someone else, blame someone else, who do you really feel negative emotions toward? Yourself.

Body Chemistry

When you go on medication for depression, it's hard because there is some physiological rebellion going on in your body. Even though, in many cases, the medication is treating a malfunction, such as certain electrical impulses or neurons in your brain that aren't making connections, your body is used to that. It is not used to the medication.

Many times, what is going to happen is that your body is going to rebel against the medication. You will be fine for two weeks or a month, and then all of a sudden your body says, "I don't like this anymore." That can happen anytime, but typically it's between two months and a year.

There's no easy way to get your body's chemistry in line. As you go through this medication adjustment, you become psychologically frustrated. Then you may think the medication isn't working. The main thing is you really have to be patient. It's surprising how once you get the combination of a mood stabilizer, an antidepressant, or something that works for anxiety, you will suddenly feel in control of your emotions and behaviors. What you start feeling is what puts stops into the negativity.

I used to have a temper. I would have temper tantrums that could last for three days. After starting meds, if I encountered a situation in which I was upset, of course I would begin going through all the lovely parts of one of my temper outbursts. You know, dark thoughts like "exterminate the human race" type of thing. But after a minute or two, I could say, "Wait, let's logically look at this. What's happening?"

Believe me, prior to medication, I never did that. I got angry, possibly broke things, threatened to do harm to people, and in my younger days, did do harm to people. Then I would go into a state of depression, a flat line, and then I'd come back. It was pretty much a ritual with me. In fact, you could count on it like clockwork.

Now I'm at a different level of getting emotionally well, and the physical end is beginning to take hold. I'm getting my body back into shape and it feels good. Of course, the process takes a bit of time, six months to a year as I said earlier. The point is that I'm at a different level now, and it feels good.

CHAPTER NINE
INTERMITTENT RAGE EPISODES

[SK]

Many bipolar patients experience intermittent rage episodes, as Keith described in the previous chapter. A percentage of people with Tourette syndrome and ADHD suffer from rage episodes as well.

Although rather mysterious, rage episodes—sometimes called limbic rage or temporal lobe syndrome—appear to be of two varieties:

1. Those associated with frustration, anxiety, and response to the word no.

2. Those which share some characteristics of seizures.

Most bipolar patients experience the type of rage attacks associated with a buildup of anxiety and frustration, often in response to not getting their way or things not going well for them. This is as true of children as of adults. If a child with bipolar characteristics is told no, he or she will often experience a buildup of anxiety and frustration so severe that property damage results and other people are in danger of getting hurt. Likewise, adults who are frustrated by things not going well, as described by Keith in the previous chapter, can experience anxiety, frustration, and then rage.

Often the bipolar patient does not remember the details of the incident and reports being unable to control the outburst, although he is vaguely aware that it is occurring. These rage attacks can last for hours and even days. They often cause tremendous damage to property and relationships. Once over, the patient's mood becomes more mellow for a period—until the anxiety and frustration again build to the point of rage.

It is difficult for family members to understand rage episodes because each event is so unpredictable. An incident that at one time will not incite a rage will do so at another time. Therefore, family members tiptoe around, waiting for the volcano to erupt.

In adult bipolars, alcohol will very often incite rage episodes. Perhaps this is because the "stop" is removed and the bipolar's underlying anxiety, frustration, and anger are allowed to explode without any way to logically process situations in a reality-based manner.

A drunk bipolar can be like a raging bull, becoming extremely angry about things that were not issues in the past. Abuse is often the result of this type of rage, which is terrifying and confusing to family members.

The intermittent rage episodes associated with Tourette syndrome and severe ADHD can be similar to those described above. However, there is also a very different type of rage seen in some of these patients and probably in some bipolar patients as well.

This other type of rage is not necessarily associated with anything in the environment, although it can be. It can happen because the weather is rainy outside or something is lost or some other very insignificant event occurs that is out of proportion for the degree of anger exhibited.

This type if rage is more characteristic of a seizure and can be broken down into five distinct phases.

1. *The aura (prodroma).* The patient can feel that a rage attack is coming on. Often the patient will express fear or dread. "Please help me, I'm going to freak out!"

2. *A change in physical appearance, especially the eyes.* The eyes become rather blank. There is a primitive characteristic to the patient, who can no longer be reached.

3. *The actual rage attack.* During the attack, the patient is out of control. Often this requires that the patient be held down or restrained in some way to avoid hurting self or others. The patient has tremendous strength at this time, which can make restraint difficult. This phase can last for hours.

4. *The twilight stage.* During this stage, the patient frequently sleeps, having become completely exhausted from raging.

5. *Confusion/disorientation/denial/remorse.* After sleeping, the patient is often confused and disoriented. The patient may have no memory of the attack. When informed, there is often denial, more confusion, and tremendous remorse over the incident.

Many patients with this type of seizure-like rage have negative electroencephalograms (EEGs), while a small percent have positive studies. This type of rage is thought to be associated with changes in the primitive part of the brain, the limbic system, which is the very core or center of the brain, and some EEGs do not pick up signals that deep. Many parents who are hoping for a positive EEG, so they have documentation of the problem, are disappointed to be told their child has a negative study. Because of the severity of these episodes, it is not surprising that parents want to know what is causing them.

I feel this type of rage is somewhat like a dream to the patient. They are hoping it isn't true, but when they learn it is, they are embarrassed, horrified, and guilt-ridden. They are also extremely frightened by the loss of control they have experienced.

Many people with rage isolate. They fear they will suffer a rage attack in public, where the embarrassment and potential for criminal activity is great. Many try desperately to control the rage, but often find control impossible.

Some people with intermittent rage are fascinated with fire. I believe this is especially true for those who suffer the seizure-like rage episodes.

Strobe lights and many other light-associated activities, like some computer games, are known to cause seizures in those who are seizure-prone.

I believe (and this is my theory only) that fascination with fire makes sense for rage-prone patients, especially children. Fires are often relatively accessible and strobe lights are not. The act of staring at a fire can bring on a seizure or a rage attack. This affords the patient an element of control over an otherwise uncontrollable aspect of behavior. The patient gains control over *when* the rage attack will occur. Parents have reported that children who stare at fires will often have a rage attack shortly thereafter. Perhaps the behavior of staring at a fire in a child who is prone to rage attacks is one element of control children can gain over the monster inside.

It is imperative to get the rage under control immediately. It is important to find a doctor who understands rage and can successfully treat it. It is rare for rage to be controlled without medication. Generally, mood stabilizers and/or antianxiety medications are most effective in treating rage.

Intermittent rage episodes are more common than people realize, yet the literature on the topic is sadly limited and generally clinical. These episodes are responsible for more broken lives and hearts than most care to admit. By understanding their existence, we can begin to better deal with the serious consequences of untreated rage.

[KC]

Psychological Programming

After getting your body chemistry in better shape, the next thing to tackle is your psychological programming. To be the way you were—depressed, angry, anxious—has been an ingrained part of your psyche. It was in mine for about forty years.

Even after the meds start taking effect, you will still psychologically rebel at times, not want to take your medication, or catch yourself going into depressed states. The meds are not a save-all solution. They will put some stops in, but they will not make you better. You have to do that!

You can go to every "Dr. Feel Good" in the world, but guess what? It's not going to make your life better. It will give you some tools to cope better, but you are still going to have your ups and you are still going to have your downs.

Now, I don't like being aggravated, but it was what I was used to. The littlest thing pushed me right over the edge, and that's the way I operated. To become different took time, a long time.

You see, in a way, as you start to get better, you sit on the fence. You can go in either direction, and hopefully you will want to return to the more emotionally stable side.

Perhaps the best way to describe it is that you are walking down a road. On the right-hand side of the road is the proper way, the way you really want to live. On this side, you are emotionally stable and you can cope with just about anything that is thrown at you.

But, then of course, there is the left-hand side—the way you are used to. You know you can go over to that side. You know you can get angry, you can drink and abuse your family, you can vent, rant, rave, and be negative. That's what you know best, because that's what you've done the longest.

Unfortunately, it's going to take some time to stay consistently on the right-hand side, but the reward when you do is worth the effort it took.

Oh sure, you might weave all over the road as you try to get from the old negative side to the new positive, but you can stay on the road. You'll probably weave toward one shoulder of the road and then to the other side. Then you'll be able to drive down the middle of the road for a while. You'll have to talk to yourself and keep encouraging yourself so you can recognize where you are. You can ask yourself, "Am I on the right side or left side right now? Am I on the side I want to be on?" Keep yourself in check and keep heading forward.

One weird thing that happens as you are doing this physiological change, along with the psychological change, is that your body and your mind will not want you in that stable place. In fact, they protest early and often. Your body has only known how to be whacked and doesn't know what to do with the change. Your mind is accustomed to constant chaos and is often bored with stability.

Friends When You Change

Another weird thing that happened to me concerned my old drinking buddies. When I became more emotionally healthy, all my so-called friends, come to find out, were a bunch of kooks too. They sure didn't like the idea that I was stable. They didn't like the idea that I was trying to make a family work. Well, that infuriated me. Yes, I let it bother me. But that's consistent with how I've always been. And, of course, that's the way they wanted me to be.

So the issue then becomes, who are your friends? Are they other people with issues similar to yours? You know the old adage about people flocking together. Wouldn't real friends be happy for you and encourage you to get healthy and improve your family life? I think so.

There is a saying that people can turn on you when they just want to be like you. When you change, often you have an effect on them, but you can also be foreign to them. When my friends saw my improvement, they saw I was no longer like them. Then I had to deal with my reaction to them.

It was hard because I could have said, "This guy is an SOB and I won't continue to see him." That was my choice to make, after all.

But some of these people had been my friends for fifteen to forty years. The best way to understand their behavior is to remind yourself that their reactions are not your fault. Some people and circumstances have brought changes into your life, and your friends have decided to turn away because of those changes. You didn't turn on your friends. You turned toward a better, healthier life for you.

Your friends didn't help you with your mess during all those years. The new people you're involved with—your spouse, children, and family who have finally gotten fed up and gotten it through your head that you need treatment—are the people who are really concerned about you and who have really helped you.

I look back and see how my friends gave me a bad time when I tried to improve. They bantered me with, "Is that your wife talking?" I countered back with, "You bet it's my wife talking, and I'm a better person because of her."

As I got healthier, it felt strange because I began enjoying family instead of experiencing the old feeling that they were draining me. I enjoyed quiet times rather than going after those bouts of seeking adrenaline.

I said in an earlier chapter that I brought consistency to my friends—I might either blow my cork or be fun and full of jokes, but they could count on me to have a few drinks and spend the evening listening or joking, whichever happened.

The hardest thing for me with my friends disappearing was that I felt abandoned again, the way I had felt abandoned as a child. It felt like they really didn't care after all. Now, I'm not so sure that's the issue—them leaving because they stopped caring. I think they always cared, but they're just not used to the new, improved me. They surrounded me when I was like them, but when I changed, they didn't stay with me because I was no longer like them.

When I was single, I got involved with a group of middle-aged people. It was quite interesting how they operated. They all had issues similar to mine. Many had drinking problems, many had relationship problems, and they all banded together because they were all the same. I had a little more of a moral concept and got out of that group.

One thing I noticed is that when I came out of the drinking subculture, I lost a few friends. I admit I had a drinking problem because I was self-medicating. But I'm away from that now and doing well.

The takeaway from all of this is that if you want to get better, you cannot let friends who don't want to see you get better rule your life. It's hard because so many times I think of my friends and the things they say about my family and my wife. I suppose in a sense they are jealous. My friends wanted things the way they were—me the way I was. I was dependent on them, and they were dependent on me. We had this co-dependent relationship going.

Now I'm a totally different being who is trying to live a different life. People notice and tell me that I'm different, not the same. One of the best things about it is I can say, "Yes, I know I'm different. And there's not much you can do to change me back. I feel much better about myself, and I hope you feel better about me too." And I leave it at that. If people are your true friends, they will continue to want to be part of your life.

When you change your thoughts, you set off a series of other changes. You change your behavior. You change your attitude. You change your friends. Sometimes change involves giving up the old. That can be painful, but what you get in return can be much better than what you gave up. Don't be afraid to change.

[SK]

The major reason change is difficult is because of what Keith describes above in such great detail.

Our comfort zone in any situation is known as homeostasis. Homeostasis can be simply defined as the normal state of any system. A family is a system and therefore finds comfort with homeostasis. Anytime change occurs, homeostasis is disrupted and the entire system must change. Thus, change requires a great deal of courage, because the system is seeking to return to the prior state of familiar homeostasis. With any permanent change, the person must understand that there is going to be fear of the unknown. The past is the comfort zone that is familiar and safe for everyone involved. When there is change, unfamiliar behavior creates fear for the entire system. Familiar behavior that has been established is now being changed and people expect the familiar behavior to continue in the same pattern as before. When homeostasis is disrupted, other people within the system resist the change. They attempt to return the system to the familiar patterns of the prior system because that is comfortable and safe for them. Permanent change creates loss. This can include loss of friends, substances, rituals, comfort levels, and homeostasis. These losses are extremely significant. Therefore, when a person is changing, a great deal of outside encouragement and support are essential for success.

People change for three reasons.

1. The old way is no longer working.

2. They have learned a new/better way of doing things.

3. They've experienced crisis (hit bottom).

Of the three, crisis is the most motivating. However, as you can see from Keith's journey, the other two motivators are powerful as well. Many times, all three motivators work together to bring about change.

It took a great deal of courage for Keith to step out of his comfort zone and make healthy changes.

Chapter Ten
Transition to Health

[SK]

Generic Medications

Many of my patients have reported that generic medications do not have the same effect on them as the brand medications do. Generics, although more economical, are often inconsistent in the dosage each pill delivers. While generics are generally fine for most people, I have seen people with Tourette syndrome, ADHD, bipolar disorder, and other mood disorders who do not respond as well. It is my feeling that because of the imbalance in brain chemistry of these patients, they require absolute consistency in dosing. Any change in this consistency can cause the generic medication to be ineffective.

If this happens to you or your child, be aware of it and ask your doctor to check the "do not substitute" box on the written prescription form. This will require the pharmacy to fill the prescription with the brand-name medication rather than the generic. The prescription will likely cost more, but it is definitely worth it to assure the medication works. The same may be true of all medications, including antibiotics and medications not associated with brain functioning.

The inconsistency of generic medications can cause much questioning about medications and their effects in general. If you have just refilled a prescription with a generic that does not work, and the drug had previously been effective as a brand-name product, please consider trying the brand name again before changing to a different medication.

Antibiotics
I have noticed that when patients are taking antibiotics, their antidepressants become much less effective. Over the course of my practice, I have seen patient after patient complain of depression worsening while on antibiotics. Patients who are clinically improving from depression and subsequently begin a course of antibiotic treatment often experience an increase in depression symptoms. This confuses and frustrates them because they cannot figure out why they have become so depressed again.

Knowing that antibiotics can make antidepressants less effective is valuable information. If it is explained to the patient that the increased depression will abate after the antibiotics are discontinued, the patient is relieved.

If antibiotic treatment is anticipated to be long term, the patient can contact the prescribing psychiatrist or physician to inquire about obtaining additional help with the depression during the course of the antibiotic treatment.

Medications are often a critical piece in transitioning to health, and now you have more information to help make the transition.

[KC]

Mental Conditioning
It's been my experience that what we focus on continually will grow. What we do not focus on will eventually diminish and die. This includes dark thoughts, anger, and any other negative thoughts or behavior like drinking or drug abuse. The less we do the negative and the more we do other things, the more likely it is that the behavior that we wish to change will eventually disappear.

Sometimes people can say or do the dumbest things. For many years prior to treatment, I felt disappointed with the human race for not seeing my side. People disappointed me. But then the light bulb went on and I realized I could manage the trigger by either doing my breathing or having good thoughts. I just had to tell myself that the current time was going to be difficult, extremely difficult, but I could handle it.

I've proved it in my own life. I used to think dark thoughts 98 percent of the time. I still think them. However, something new I'm doing is not reinforcing the negative.

As I'm moving along and thinking negative thoughts or thoughts of hopelessness or despair (which still happens 80 percent of the time), I catch myself shaking my head and saying, "Wait a minute. Do not think about that. What else can I think about?" And I'll get a thought about how to improve something at work or a way to improve my home life. I may even think of ways to help people.

By now you may be thinking, "So what? You're just thinking a little bit about it." But, you see, the beauty is that awareness allows for choices. I have found that I have a choice to think one thought over another.

Let's say I cut the thought process of negative thinking down to 60 percent of the time. That means I'm now thinking good things 40 percent of the time, or twice as much. Eventually, those extra twenty percentage points will override even more of the negative. Change is slow, but gradual, positive change is still positive change.

I believe people, as a whole, like instant gratification. They want to see quick results for any effort, but that's not always possible.

I have noticed that with the dark thoughts, even after learning how to control them, it still takes a tremendous amount of energy to get the brain going positive. But I don't give up working on stopping them.

[SK]

This process can be compared to dieters who are losing weight. While they often want to lose weight fast and may temporarily succeed with crash diets, permanent weight loss is usually only possible through slow, permanent dietary changes. These gradual, positive changes are often the most effective and lasting.

1. Instant gratification can be achieved with crash diets, but it is extremely rare for that weight loss to be permanent.

2. Although frustrating, the gradual positive changes very often lead to permanent weight loss.

[KC]

Mental Workout

One time, about three weeks after a truly manic state that lasted for two days, I found that my mind was coming back into better shape. About two weeks after the manic state, I experienced a minor manic episode. I was able to defuse it pretty quickly, but afterward I noticed that before the manic state, which started in the early evening, I had not eaten. I feel certain my blood sugar levels were starting to go awry or possibly my body was just hungry. In the past, skipping meals could be a form of a trigger in me.

It's become more apparent to me that after controlling the manic states, I am better able to interact with people in a positive manner, even causing people to laugh—especially family members.

Bipolars can experience a rather unfortunate pattern with people at times. Outwardly in public, they are jovial, appearing almost happy. But in private, the person their loved ones usually see feels the pain and despair so commonly associated with the disorder.

It is interesting that you can be jovial and actually quite fun around strangers while you use your family members as a toxic waste dump. As for me, I could handle being happy or joking around other people because, in a sense, I was pretty much fooling them with my ability to appear to be control.

I had heard you can never change a first impression. So if I came across as an in-control, happy person who was confident, that's how people saw me versus how I really was inside—very weak, very frightened, and sometimes acting very ignorant.

Sometimes it may be more effective for the bipolar person to adopt a stop mechanism rather than one that replaces the negative thoughts with positive thoughts. Sometimes it was more effective for me to just stop the negative thoughts and not worry about thinking anything else. As one therapist told me, it was like I had blinders on. Like a horse, I could see what was in front of me, but not what was around me.

Looking at what was in front of me was a distinct habit I had. When I looked at what was ahead of me, I either dwelled on the negative behavior or obsessed about the anticipatory anxiety. Then I looked at everything around me, including at the fact I had a lot of literally dormant resources around me.

[SK]

I believe this anticipatory anxiety is the huge problem for many bipolar patients and is what prevents many from enjoying the present moment. When they finally get focused into the *now*, they are surprised and relieved to find that it is all they have to think and worry about. It is then that they truly begin to "smell the flowers" and enjoy life to the fullest.

[KC]

Sarah already talked about how bipolars are creative and intelligent. I agree we can think quite quickly, making racing thoughts a potential problem. But one of the issues is that bipolars have to be driven to a manic state. It is when you come down from a manic state that your best brilliance appears. I've seen that pattern most of my adult life.

[SK]

The moments of true brilliance and creativity are the main reasons many bipolars resist treatment. They often lose this brilliance when medication levels their moods and the manic state leaves. This cuts down tremendously on creativity and sometimes motivation, which can be a great loss both personally and professionally. Many bipolars would rather suffer the pain of manic and depressive states than lose their window of brilliance, especially after so many years of having had it. That decision, of course, has a negative impact on their relationships. Again, many brilliant, creative people have sacrificed their personal lives and themselves in pursuit of this window of (manic) greatness.

[KC]

Prior to treatment, I used to have a one-day cycle of rage followed by total adrenaline-seeking, furniture-breaking release. After therapy, the cycle was down to once a week. After treatment with mood stabilizers and antidepressants, the cycle is about every three weeks. I've definitely been able to be happier and more relaxed.

Now I can tell when my body is itching for a manic state and I literally have to fight to prevent it.

One thing I notice is that after all the therapy, after all the medications, I still have to do the work to be completely aware of what's around me instead of putting on my blinders and looking straight ahead.

Certain issues I dealt with for so many years, such as misplacing or losing things, are no longer issues. I can actually remember where things are. I get maybe ten seconds of "Where did they go?" Then I'll look around and remember where they are.

If you live with someone who suffers from the losing and misplacing syndrome, you should know that many of us have obsessive-compulsive issues. If our stuff gets moved, we get upset.

For me, it's helped a lot to get organized and put things in one place. It gives me a form of mental stability.

Mental stability is a gift to a bipolar. What appear to be small things to most people (thinking positive thoughts, making healthy choices, learning to stop and think about where things are), can be life-changing for those who've spent their lives living with dark thoughts, engaging in self-defeating behavior like mutilation or negative self-talk, and reacting with mania or depression because something isn't as or where they expected.

Remember change comes slowly, and it doesn't always take a straight path. But change does come, and with it comes the gradual transition to health.

SECTION TWO
CHILDHOOD NEUROLOGICAL DISORDERS, INCLUDING TOURETTE SYNDROME

Chapter Eleven
Tourette Syndrome in Childhood

[SK]

Tourette syndrome is becoming more common, although often not diagnosed. Getting a proper diagnosis is the first step for families in handling many behavioral and medical aspects associated with this condition.

Identifying Tourette syndrome, recognizing its effect on the family, and having the expertise to effectively intervene is very important for a family therapist and other professionals.

Today, Tourette syndrome is recognized as a neurological disorder with associated behavior aberrations. It's the associated behaviors that often send patients to a mental health professional, so it's beneficial for the professional to recognize the signs of Tourette syndrome and refer the patient for the appropriate care.

Psychotherapy is essential in helping the family deal with Tourette syndrome.

Tourette Journey

I'm going to take you on a journey into the mind, body, and very being of a person with Tourette syndrome.

One day all is well. You feel in control of your mind and body. But on the first day of the journey, you find your body is doing things you cannot control and your mind is thinking thoughts you don't want to think.

Your face grimaces and twitches. You feel a compelling need to run, to hit your friends, to touch and retouch an object an even number of times. For some strange reason, you want to smell dirty socks.

Next, you are spitting and swearing—two things you've never done in public (or in private for that matter).

You have become a slave to an uncontrollable force within your mind and body that has literally stripped you of your free will, of your very being.

Your feelings vacillate between being ashamed and not caring. With great concentration, you may be able to control your body movements and thought processes for a little while, much in the same way a person controls the urge to cough or sneeze, but you always know that sometime soon the strange power will win the battle over you.

Are you going crazy? You may fear so, and others may well agree. If you are very fortunate, you may seek help from a professional who recognizes Tourette syndrome and can properly diagnose and treat you.

If you are more unfortunate, you will suffer for years, wondering what is wrong with you while you, your family, your friends, and all of society think you have lost self-control.

You are the proverbial square peg in the round hole. The world expects you to conform and interprets your invisible disability as rudeness, egocentricity, or insanity.

As we conclude our journey into the world of Tourette syndrome, let's ponder how you would react to this strange new way of being. Let's also leave with a desire to learn more about this disorder so you may begin to understand the problems encountered by people who live with Tourette syndrome every day.

Education helps us understand. Understanding helps us accept and embrace people with Tourette syndrome into our lives and into our hearts.

Diagnosis

Tourette syndrome typically has an onset between ages two and twenty. It has a waxing and waning course. For a diagnosis of Tourette syndrome to be made, both a motor and vocal tic must be present for a period of at least one year. Tics can be difficult to identify as one tic is replaced by another and the severity changes. Shoulder shrugging may be exchanged for face grimacing or eye blinking. Many patients become good at camouflaging tics. A vocal tic can be camouflaged as an allergy symptom. Also, tics can be suppressed for a short while, but they are not voluntary. Suppression takes great concentration and/or effort, and after a period of suppression, tics are generally worse.

Tics that are camouflaged are especially difficult to identify unless one is quite familiar with the disorder. This is especially true of vocal tics. People with throat-clearing or sniffing tics often camouflage them as allergy-type problems. Vocal tics include sounds that are not recognized as words. They are repetitious in nature and vary in intensity. They can be as soft as a whisper or as loud and explosive as a scream. They can include barking, spitting, humming, throat-clearing, grunting, snorting, squeaking, or any other meaningless, repetitive sound. Coprolalia is involuntary swearing and is considered to be a vocal tic.

Motor tics are often more difficult to camouflage. However, the shoulder shrugging, eye blinking and lip licking can be mistaken for normal developmental stages, especially if the child is active. While the child's tics may be benign forms of overactivity, the child could be displaying hidden forms of motor tics.

In transient tic disorder of childhood, there is a shorter duration and absence of vocal tics. While similar to Tourette syndrome, transient tic disorder is a milder form that generally disappears in less than one year.

Motor tics include involuntary movements of any muscle, ranging from sudden, rapid, jerking motions to slow, stretching movements. Like vocal tics, these movements are purposeless, repetitive, and involuntary. Some examples are yawning motions (mouth opening), rolling head movements, contortions of the face, protrusions of the tongue, stretching movements, blinking or upward glancing of the eyes, shrugging of shoulders, or licking of lips.

Many people are unaware of internal tics. Burping, belching, and feeling an urgency to urinate are a few internal tics. It is especially difficult for others to understand these tics. A child who is constantly belching is soon told to stop. People simply do not understand the child has an internal tic that is part of Tourette syndrome.

Coprolalia is probably the best-known symptom of Tourette syndrome. It is the involuntary vocalization of swear words. While present in less than half of Tourette patients, coprolalia is certainly the most profound and fascinating symptom of the disorder. It is therefore often depicted when Tourette syndrome is shown in movies, documentaries or television shows.

Those afflicted with coprolalia are often frustrated by the inability of others to understand these words are involuntary. Many employers do not wish to hire a person who swears on a regular and involuntary basis. That often limits employment to jobs that are hidden away from the public. Coprolalia limits its victims in all aspects of their lives, from going to the grocery store to earning a living.

Sadly, because coprolalia is so often featured as the primary symptom of Tourette syndrome, many people believe its presence is needed to make a diagnosis. People are often misdiagnosed because of the absence of this symptom. Because coprolalia is noted in less than half of Tourette syndrome cases, this misrepresentation can do a disservice to the majority of patients without it who are struggling to be correctly diagnosed and understood.

Interestingly, tics, including coprolalia, often vanish when the patient is in a state of deep concentration. A musician playing in the orchestra, who otherwise demonstrates severe Tourette symptoms, is without them while playing drums on stage. Likewise, a surgeon who is operating has steady hands during surgical procedures, though his tics cause significant hand motion at other times. This is one of the great mysteries of Tourette syndrome.

In Tourette syndrome, there is a problem with inhibition control of the mind and body. Inhibition control is a very important part of human development and behavior.

Keith talks about "stops" being lost in bipolar patients. In Tourette syndrome patients, there are also lost "stops." Inhibition control is minimal or lost, resulting in body movements and vocal sounds that make little sense. There are generally a number of these body movements and vocalizations (or tics) present at the same time.

There is another component to loss of inhibition control that involves the mind. In these patients, and especially children, whatever is in the mind is on the lips. With decreased stops, it is common for Tourette patients to say what they are thinking, sometimes whether it is appropriate or not. For example, we may think a person is wearing an ugly dress. We would never tell the person what we're thinking about the dress. However, a Tourette child may say something like, "That is the ugliest dress I have ever seen." They may manifest their thoughts in other ways as well. For example, if they are thinking about throwing an eraser across a classroom, they have great difficulty stopping themselves from doing so.

As the Tourette child matures, behaviors like those described above become more and more unacceptable, which creates more embarrassment. People find it difficult to understand that hurtful or inappropriate comments and behaviors are not done purposefully. Thus, Tourette patients can lose friends and respect from others quickly.

Tourette syndrome is more common in males than females. It is a genetic neurological condition that is present in every race, region, and social status in the world.

Associated Behavior

There are other behaviors associated with Tourette syndrome. These can include depression, obsessive-compulsive disorder, anxiety, phobias, behavior problems, low frustration tolerance level, mood swings, intermittent rage episodes, short attention span, hyperactivity, learning problems, and dyslexia. There can be associated problems with normal socialization.

Depression is associated with Tourette syndrome. It is often difficult to determine whether this is the result of daily problems encountered by the patient, or if it is an additional manifestation. Regardless of the cause, depression is an additional consideration in the successful management of the Tourette syndrome patient.

A frequent feature of Tourette syndrome is a somewhat strange form of obsessive-compulsive behavior. When severe, compulsive behaviors can be extremely debilitating. Many children lick their lips until they bleed. Some often hit themselves (some experts consider this a tic rather than an obsessive-compulsive behavior). Others like to smell unusual things like people's feet, spoiled food, and even dead animals.

Compulsive behaviors begin with an intense interest in something that gradually progresses to a compulsion. One child who became interested in history could name every president of the United States in order and also name each president's opponent in each election—and he was only nine years old. A compulsion like this can become an asset. However, many parents of Tourette syndrome children tire of the subject matter long before the child does.

Some bizarre behaviors other patients have manifested include trying to see how close to the edge of the roof they could get (without falling off), picking off wallpaper, trying to open the car door and jump out while the car is in motion, unusual interest in fires, biting on shirt collars, and fascination with knives and scissors. Many of these behaviors have an obsessive-compulsive component to them, and some of them have a dark nature.

Raising a Tourette syndrome child is a challenge that can never be done "by the book." On a daily basis, the child is often overwhelmed by demands to control himself, to which the answer is, "I can't." If teachers and other adults do not understand the disorder, they will expect the Tourette child to behave like other children. The inability to control tics and behavior often upsets this child tremendously. A child with Tourette syndrome will often seem oblivious to any type of traditional disciplinary technique. Since he usually has a well-developed conscience, the consequences of an inability to conform to expectations can be severe.

Behavior modification, positive reinforcement, and time-outs are generally the most effective disciplinary strategies when dealing with a Tourette child.

Tourette children have difficulty taking breaks from tasks. Once these children begin to tell a story or play a game, it is important for them to finish. Though this behavior is sometimes mistaken for being demanding, often it occurs because the child cannot let the thought go until it is finished. Trying to rush the child to the end of the story or game will cause frustration and can trigger a temper outburst. A story may be repeated again and again in a compulsive way. It is important to be aware of time limitations and remind the child there may not be enough time to finish. A timer can be used as a warning device.

Sometimes medication can help with behavior problems. However, because of the ever-changing, waxing and waning course of the disorder, medications may have to be changed to accommodate new symptoms. This can be extremely difficult and frustrating.

Psychotherapy cannot cure Tourette syndrome. However, it can help with self-esteem issues. Because of the inability to control body movements and vocal noises, the child often has problems fitting in. Add learning problems, anxiety, and depression, and it is easy to understand the need for work on self-esteem.

A Tourette patient can teach a therapist about the courage required to face a day with the debilitating symptoms of Tourette syndrome. Helping the child through these difficulties can be a positive learning experience for the therapist as new strategies are developed to help the child cope in a world that he or she does not understand. With every victory, the bond between therapist and patient becomes closer and the case more rewarding

Attention deficit hyperactivity disorder (ADHD) is very commonly associated with Tourette syndrome. For that reason, it is discussed in extensive detail below. ADHD has four components.

1. *Inattention and distractibility*—Hyperactive children have difficulty concentrating and paying attention. The more boring the subject matter, the more difficulty they have paying attention.

2. *Hyperactivity with Overarousal and excessive activity*—Hyperactive children are very restless and overactive. They are very dramatic. They have trouble sitting still for long periods of time. They experience emotions, such as happiness, anger, sadness, and frustration, more often and more intensely than other children their age.

3. *Impulsiveness and Difficulty with rules and rewards*—Hyperactive children have problems following rules. This is because they have difficulty thinking before acting. They also may not benefit from past experiences. These children have difficulty working toward long-term goals and instead require repeated short-term pay-offs.

4. *Emotional Instability*—Hyperactive children are emotionally unstable. They have quick tempers and low frustration tolerance levels. They cry easily and have more ups and downs than other children.

Because of their similar natures, it is frequently difficult (sometimes impossible) to differentiate a severe case of ADHD from one of Tourette syndrome—and often the label is merely academic. It is obvious that one disorder enhances the behavior manifestations of the other.

The onset of ADHD may precede the onset of Tourette syndrome by approximately two years.

In addition to problems with ADHD, many Tourette patients suffer from learning disabilities. These include problems with written language, arithmetic, and reading. Sometimes treating the ADHD with stimulants will improve the learning problems, but can make the tics worse.

Family Issues

Tourette syndrome can have a tremendous impact on a family. A child with Tourette syndrome can cause problems between spouses, among siblings, and with extended family members. Because of Tourette syndrome's tendency to be inherited, often another family member has the disorder, and the two patients have problems between themselves as well as with other family members.

Unaffected siblings of the Tourette child can often be overlooked. They generally do not receive the amount of attention given the child with Tourette syndrome. This can create additional problems within the family. Sometimes the sibling may begin to exhibit signs of Tourette syndrome. It can be difficult to determine whether these behaviors appear because the sibling desires more attention, is simply imitating the affected sibling, or is experiencing real manifestations of the Tourette syndrome gene.

Often before a diagnosis is made, the blame game is played among family members. It goes something like, "If only his father weren't so hard on him, he'd be okay," or "If only his sister didn't pick on him, he'd be okay," or "If only we'd spent more time with him, he'd be okay," or "If only his mother weren't so easy on him, he'd be okay," or "If only he didn't play so many video games, he'd be okay." Of course, the end result of the blame game is guilt, and guilt isn't healthy.

Often families change things in a desperate attempt to fix the child with Tourette syndrome. Mom may quit her job and spend more time with the child. Sister might be told not to pick on him so much. Dad goes easier on him and Mom is harder on him. His video game playing time is limited to one hour per day. He is taken to the amusement park or the ball park, and is enrolled in lessons of some kind. Yet the behavior continues.

The reason for the continuation of the behavior is that everything has been addressed except the real problem. The real problem is neurologically based, and until that aspect of the disorder is understood and addressed, very little improvement can be expected.

Once it is understood that the child suffers from a neurological disorder, the blame game can end. It is often a great relief to a family that has been suffering and searching for answers. There can also be a tremendous sense of guilt. There are two components of guilt.

1. The parents feel guilt because they produced an imperfect child. One parent may blame the other if it is felt the other parent passed on the Tourette syndrome gene.

2. Parents may also experience guilt because they have been insensitive to the fact that the child's behavior was based on a neurological disorder and could not be controlled. They have sent him to his room for all that twitching, or for being disruptive at the dinner table, and there was no way he could have changed those behaviors.

Parents may also feel a sense of frustration and failure. Nothing has worked with this child. Therefore, they feel they have failed. Standard measures of discipline generally do not work well with the Tourette child.

Parents of only children with Tourette syndrome may experience more pronounced feelings of failure because they have no basis for comparison. Thus they either believe all children are as difficult as theirs or that they are grossly ineffective parents.

When one of these disorders first appears in a family, there's confusion and frustration. The sooner the proper diagnosis is made, the sooner everyone can begin the healing process of turning black and white into gray.

Chapter Twelve
Attention Deficit Disorder

[SK]

Many patients who suffer from bipolar disorder or Tourette syndrome also have a history of ADHD or ADD. The onset of ADHD or ADD is earlier than either of the other disorders. Therefore, a patient may already be dealing with this diagnosis when evaluated for either bipolar disorder or Tourette syndrome. Because of its common co-occurrence, ADHD and ADD are discussed in detail below.

There are people who have ADHD with the H (hyperactivity), and those who have ADD with no H (without hyperactivity). The people with the H are the ones who are generally noticed in school. They are throwing erasers across the room and *always* causing trouble. Those without the H rarely get noticed—they slip through the cracks in the system. They are the quiet students sitting in the back of the classroom, daydreaming or staring out the window, not hearing what the teacher is saying.

It doesn't matter whether you're talking about ADHD or ADD; individuals with either diagnosis almost always have difficulty organizing and completing their work.

Important Signs of ADHD and ADD:

There are four characteristics associated with attention deficit disorder. They are inattention, impulsivity, hyperactivity and emotional instability.

Inattention:

One of the most prominent symptoms of ADD and ADHD is inattention. These people are not listening to what is being said because they are either daydreaming or creating chaos. Any unexpected interruption causes them to get off track and then have difficulty returning attention to their task. As students, they often put off completing overwhelming assignments like term papers until the last minute and sometimes do not finish them. This procrastination is sometimes overcome by an adrenaline rush which acts as a "stimulant" at the last minute. The student is motivated to finish the term paper in one evening, often spending many hours. If ADD or ADHD continues into adulthood, difficulty sitting still in meetings or finishing work projects often replace these childhood characteristics.

Organization is also difficult. Children have backpacks and desks crammed with papers and adults have drawers stuffed with important paperwork, mail and various other items. Searching for lost papers and other items causes frustration and time management problems for person who suffers from ADD or ADHD. Sometimes finished homework assignments are lost in the chaos of messy desks or back-packs and are never turned in for credit.

Communication is difficult with the ADD or ADHD patient. It is important to eliminate distractions, such as the TV and use clear, specific language when communicating with them. Ask for confirmation of what was said to assure your communication content was understood. Sometimes it may be beneficial to write it and say it but be specific!

Learning problems are often present with ADD and ADHD. These can include dyslexia and others, but difficulty with math is most common. As adults, this progresses to difficulty balancing the checkbook.

Impulsivity:

> People with ADD or ADHD are impulsive. They act first and then think. When they become aware of the negative consequences of their actions, they often feel remorseful. They simply do not have the ability to see the consequences until *after* they act. As children, they learn by their mistakes. Frustrated parents often tire of helplessly watching them make poor decisions that lead to difficult life lessons. It is understandable that arrest records and jail time are some of the unfortunate results of impulsivity.

> There is often an excessive shift from one activity to another and a tendency to become easily bored. Variety sometimes sustains attention, but because of their short attention spans, they change from one task to another and never finish anything. They become bored with easy tasks and frustrated with difficult ones,

> Children are inpatient and when playing games they have difficulty waiting for their turns. As adults, they have difficulty standing in lines or waiting for appointments.

> Impulsive children with ADD or ADHD often speak out in class at inappropriate times. In addition, they often interrupt conversations or answer before a question is completely asked.

> Children with ADHD require more than the average amount of supervision to maintain acceptable levels of impulse control. Children with ADD are rarely noticed and learn to compensate in silence.

Hyperactivity:

> Hyperactivity is present only in those with ADHD and includes running around and climbing excessively. Children with ADHD are generally easy to identify because they are in constant motion. They are the ones

who get out of their seats and bother others. They are in perpetual motion.

People with ADHD have difficulty sleeping and are relatively active during sleep. They roll around and kick their covers (and anyone else unlucky enough to be in the bed with them).

At times those with ADD are fidgety, similar to those with ADHD. Whether in a classroom or a meeting, these are the people who are fidgeting, having trouble sitting still, and impatiently looking at the clock (or out the window). Fidgeting includes nail-biting, knuckle-cracking, feet jiggling, and other nervous body movements.

Emotional Instability:.

People with ADD and ADHD suffer from emotional instability. There is a great deal of failure and damaged self-esteem. Sensitivity to criticism develops because of honest efforts that have been adversely judged too many times. Children with ADHD grow into adults who are defensive and somewhat argumentative. Sometimes low frustration tolerance leads to angry outbursts and fights with others. Children with ADD who have not been noticed may learned to compensate for their anger and frustration. They become fearful, insecure adults unable to reach their full potential.

ADD and ADHD in Childhood:

Similar to the rest of the world, parents notice the ADHD child. Occasionally a child with ADD gets noticed because of severe problems focusing or other learning disabilities, but that is the exception. Parents generally notice children with ADHD early in childhood because of the characteristics noted below:

Early signs of ADHD can often be seen even in infancy. As a baby, the child may have cried or screamed for no apparent reason. There may have been many eating and sleeping difficulties.

As a toddler, the child may have been in perpetual motion, accident-prone, and stubborn, with frequent temper tantrums. Sometimes ADHD children can be clumsy or uncoordinated. Many are fussy eaters.

Related problems include excessive crying, uneven temperament, overall immaturity, and exaggerated emotional responses to even minor incidents. People with ADHD are generally thought to be socially, behaviorally, and cognitively at a level two-thirds of their chronological age.

Sleep patterns are frequently inconsistent. These children do not sleep long hours. They often toss and turn excessively, and have trouble shutting their minds off.

Both ADD and ADHD are genetic and likely result from imbalance of chemicals in the brain. In some cases, symptoms of ADD and ADHD continue into adulthood.

ADD and ADHD in Adults

Adult ADD and ADHD often present differently from that in children and adolescents. Adults are often misdiagnosed because that the outward symptoms of hyperactivity disappear in adults, even though the adult is restless inside. Adults are no longer in school, and it's in school that ADHD is most obvious.

Adults with ADD or ADHD are often drawn to particular careers. Their jobs reflect their abilities. They rarely sit behind a desk for eight hours a day. More likely, they will be firemen, police officers, paramedics, construction workers, airplane pilots, or in the entertainment industry. The adrenaline rush involved in these professions is a perfect fit for the ADD/ADHD patient. They also like the variety of each day. Patients often prefer working outside to working inside. They are generally happier being self-employed, if that is possible.

You and the School

Once your child is diagnosed with bipolar disorder, Tourette syndrome, ADHD, autism, dyslexia, or any other mood disorder, you will become an advocate for your child with the schools. What you know about your child's limitations can help tremendously in making the school experience pleasant for your child.

Your Child's Teacher

There are a number of things to consider regarding your child's teacher. The two most important considerations are *consistency and experience*.

The child will benefit most from a teacher who is experienced and has taught children with similar problems in the past. This is especially important if your child is not in a special education setting.

Consistency (a teacher who is there for the entire year) is extremely important, especially for accurate knowledge of how your child is progressing from the beginning of the year to the end. If a teacher has to leave for any reason, the substitute's lack of knowledge about your child can make it difficult to evaluate your child's progress..

Another reason for consistency is that it is generally difficult for these children to tolerate change. Any alteration in teaching techniques disrupts their already limited learning abilities.

When your child has a diagnosis, it is usually okay to request a particular teacher. I recommend that parents ask other parents regarding the best teacher(s) for the coming year. Parents can also go into the classroom and observe teachers' styles to see which teacher will be the best fit for their child.

Individual Education Plans (IEPs)

Many parents are unaware that any child with a diagnosis of Tourette syndrome, ADHD, many learning disabilities, or other differences is entitled to an individualized educational plan (IEP) every year. This includes a very specific assessment of your child's unique needs for school. Mandated by the Individuals with Disabilities Education Act (IDEA) of 1997, a free, appropriate public education must be offered to all students with disabilities. Although not obligatory at private schools, IEPs may be done per policy. The IEP, which is a verbal and written program tailored to the student's needs, is reviewed annually and appropriate changes are made.

An IEP is formulated from input provided by the teacher, parents, school psychologist, and others involved in the child's education. It may provide extra test time for the child or an aide for certain classes. For a Tourette child, it may provide tic breaks during parts of the day. As I already stated, IEPs are reviewed annually and revised as indicated by the child's needs.

School Difficulties Your Child Could Encounter

In school, ADD/ADHD and Tourette syndrome children may appear inattentive and talkative. They are often daydreamers and bother other classmates. They may also have sloppy handwriting, letter reversals, and reading or math weaknesses.

Often children with Tourette syndrome and/or ADHD have tremendous educational difficulties that can be resolved with a little understanding and cooperation from the school. Many times, because these children look normal, their requests for additional help go unanswered. When creating an IEP, their limitations can be addressed and needed changes can be made to help them succeed.

Here are some simple solutions to problems your child may encounter. These can be presented to the school either personally or through an IEP.

1. Providing extra time for students with test anxiety to take exams.

2. Giving verbal tests for Tourette students who, because of tics, find it difficult to fill in the bubbles on machine-scored test sheets. Even giving the option to simply write the letter of the correct answer can be helpful. Often filling in the bubble takes a disproportionate amount of time and concentration.

3. Assigning every other math problem in a given set for ADHD students who have trouble getting through homework assignments.

4. Turning papers sideways for math problems so the lines on the paper provide columns for the numbers.

5. Making reading windows out of index cards to assist dyslexic students in focusing.

6. Providing audio books for dyslexic students.

7. Encouraging teaches to "write it and say it" when presenting material.

8. Encouraging a positive reinforcement type of discipline system.

9. Having students with auditory processing problems or dyslexia repeat homework assignments back to the teacher before leaving for the day.

10. Allowing students to use a tape recorder rather than taking notes.

11. Allowing Tourette students to take frequent tic breaks during the day.

Many students will require IEPs that address issues other than those listed above, but they are a few of the more common ones.

Dyslexia

You may have noticed your child has certain significant talents, while having tremendous difficulties with other, comparable activities. The answer to this conundrum could be dyslexia.

My son had Tourette syndrome, but we also learned he had dyslexia. Here are some of the signs that helped us figure this out; some of these things may also apply to your child.

1. He could do mazes and word searches really well, but puzzles were a constant source of frustration for him. He had an ability to see things upside down and sideways, which was perfect for mazes and word searches. However, puzzle pieces, which require more precise directional

acuity, were totally frustrating. He would place the pieces every which way and be unable to see why they didn't fit together.

2. He had a terrific memory, which compensated for other learning problems. He knew his multiplication tables because he memorized them. However, they had no inherent meaning for him. If two times three equaled six, this was true because he had memorized it. He had no concept of it. Once I put two piles of three pennies on a table to try to explain the concept to him, and he had *no* clue.

3. He had a very difficult time learning colors. We had red days and blue days, where he'd wear the color of the day, but he still struggled. He eventually learned them, but at an older age than most other kids.

4. Directions were difficult. When he said left, he could mean right. If he said up, he could mean down. If your child has trouble with left-right, up-down, over-under, and so on, it could be the result of dyslexia or some other learning problem.

5. Small motor skills were difficult. This makes sense for a child with Tourette syndrome. The uncontrolled movements of fingers create major problems with such activities as cutting with scissors or gluing model airplanes together. The movements also make filling in answers on bubble test sheets very difficult. This is probably more related to Tourette syndrome; however, many dyslexic children have similar problems with small motor skills.

6. Difficulty buttoning and zipping. Often these children wear pants and skirts with elastic waistbands because they are unable to unzip or unbutton to use the restroom. Buttoning shirts, blouses, dresses, and jackets can also create problems.

7. Many of these children are "hyper tactile." This means their skin is overly sensitive to touch. Labels in shirts

or woolen (rough) clothing often irritate many. This can also be associated with ADHD and other neurological problems like autism.

8. Literal interpretations. Most children with Tourette/ADHD and other learning differences interpret whatever is said literally. They have difficulty with abstract thinking. To them, a broken arm is an arm that's broken off. Thus, these children have difficulty understanding many jokes. A joke like, "Why did the turtle cross the street? To get to the shell station," isn't understood. A Shell station is a gas station and doesn't have anything to do with turtles. The opposite is also true. Jokes that the child thinks are hilarious are not very funny to others.

9. Following instructions. Telling an ADD/ADHD child to clean his room may result in him going to his room and sitting there staring blankly. When you ask him why his room hasn't been cleaned, he may innocently reply, "I already cleaned it. What else am I supposed to do?" Why didn't your direction work? The child needs *specific* directions. Small, specific requests are more likely to be accomplished. A better direction is, "I would like you to go to your room and pick up the toys on the floor and then please come back for further instructions." When the child returns, you can make an additional request. Another option is to write down the instructions and say them. When a child can see what needs to be done and also hear it, he is often able to do it. With these children, write things down, say them aloud, and be specific.

10. Create structure. These children (and adults) need structure in their lives. Therefore, the more closely you can follow a daily routine, the better for your child. Try to have consistent times for going to bed and getting up in the morning. Mealtimes that are routine, quiet and relaxing are also beneficial. As mentioned in an earlier chapter, it's important to set a time for homework, but be

sure your child has a say in that decision. When the child has helped determine the homework schedule, it's easier to get cooperation.

11. Discipline. The most important aspect of discipline is something that was mentioned in an earlier chapter. Negative reinforcement (taking something away) generally does not work. Rewarding the child for doing a desired behavior is positive reinforcement and works much better. Time-outs and behavior modification can be used as well, if they are used consistently by all caregivers.

Look over this list to help you succeed in reducing frustration and accomplishing goals like homework and chores. Whether your child has been diagnosed with Tourette syndrome, ADD, ADHD, dyslexia, or a mood disorder, these ideas are worth implementing. They even work well for undiagnosed siblings.

Good Communication Is Important:

We assume everyone comes from the same reality we do. If we see a black table, we assume everyone else sees it the same. Guess what? This is absolutely *not* true!

People perceive things in many different ways. There are many different pathways sensory stimuli may take. Some people are visual; some are auditory; some are tactile. A person who is auditory has to *hear* the material in order to absorb the meaning. One who is visual has to *see* what is to be learned. The person who is tactile has to *touch* or *feel* their way to learning.

It is important to understand this when dealing with different people, especially people with ADHD and learning differences. ADHD patients tend to be extremely visual or tactile. They often have difficulty understanding verbal communication when it is not accompanied by visual or tactile instructions. For example, many couples misunderstand each other because one is visual and the other auditory. If the wife tells her husband to clean the garage, he may not hear what she said or understand it clearly. No, this is not selective hearing. When he doesn't do what she tells him, she becomes angry and frustrated and he doesn't understand why, but he's too embarrassed to say anything because she might think he's stupid.

It is possible he did not understand what she meant because she wasn't specific enough ("clean the garage" could have meant sweep it or pick up the stuff on the floor), or he may have had so many other things on his mind that her request just didn't sink in. But this failure of communication causes a real problem in many marriages. I've had enough of these couples in my office to testify to this—and they typically come see me because they're having communication problems.

This is why it is so important to understand exactly how other people in your life absorb information. One way to do this is by mirroring. The wife can ask, "What did I just ask you to do?" However, that sounds a bit demeaning. It's much safer to cover the bases of understanding—write it, say it, and be specific. Get a blackboard or a whiteboard and write simple requests on it. That way, each time the visual person passes the board, a nonthreatening reminder is seen. In the above example, if "sweep the garage" is written on the board, the visual person will be more likely to see what is written and then actually do it!

Take Time for Yourselves
It's easy to understand how demanding your life can become when raising a difficult child with a mood disorder.

It's not easy to balance a difficult child, daily living, financial stability, working, personal goals, and giving time to each other in your marriage. Your relationship might get put aside to take care of the other things you have to do.

I urge you to make time for each other. No matter what it takes, find a way to go out every week or to find a hobby you both enjoy. If you don't, you will put the quality of your relationship at risk. Your challenging child will drain you of everything you have, and you will have nothing left to give each other.

I see too many parents in my practice, good people, who put everything into their children and have nothing left for each other. When their children grow up and leave home, these parents are often strangers. The most important thing parents can do for their children is to stay in love with each other. It's difficult to do when you have a child with a mood disorder, but it is important and well worth the effort.

Behavior or Disorder?

Behavior or disorder? This question can present a confusing problem. Was your sister's rage episode because her medication dosage was off or because of unacceptable behavior? Did your son steal the final exam because of ADHD impulse control problems or was it a form of unacceptable behavior? Did your husband really mean those things he said or was it part of a manic episode?

This book is written not to provide excuses for unacceptable behavior, but to educate. When in doubt between behavior and disorder, we must assume *behavior* because the rest of society will. Sorry, but your son's teacher will not excuse his poor judgment because of his ADHD. Furthermore the police will not overlook his foolish decision to rob a convenience store in ten years. All people with mood disorders must learn to conform. This takes support, education, effort, and discipline. Is it difficult? Yes. Is it worth it? You decide.

Appendix
Questionnaire

[KC]

If you have been diagnosed with bipolar disorder, you may want to take a self-inventory with this questionnaire. In fact, you may want to take it periodically to see how you're doing.

1. Have you ever contemplated suicide? If you have, how often have you considered it, and what seems to trigger you to begin thinking about it?

2. Do you feel you have difficulties in relationships because of a negative attitude?

3. Do you enjoy activities that require extreme physical ability?

4. Do you like doing things that can demonstrate your power in one way or another?

5. Do you feel your life is out of control?

6. Do you feel that the world is wrong for you?

7. Do you habitually get angry enough to have a rage, break things, scream? If so, how often does that happen—weekly, monthly, quarterly, annually?

8. Do you think you can ever be cured of your emotional issues? Do you feel you can cure yourself?

9. Do you ever feel the need to totally isolate, just be alone for long periods of time, without any human contact?

10. Do you feel better when you are alone?

11. Has anyone in your family committed suicide? If so, how do you feel about that person? What type of impact did it have on your family?

12. Do people generally irritate you?

13. Do you have trouble standing in a line or being patient in a store when you have a problem with a retail customer in front of you?

14. Do you think you would be happier living alone?

15. Do you think a perfect job would be where you are alone to do your tasks without interruption for eight hours a day?

16. Would you rather be around machinery than people?

17. In percentages, how much of your time do you feel you spend in a depressed state? What percent of your time do you feel in the middle, "normal" area? What percent of your time do you feel euphoric or high?

18. Do you feel most people can't think as quickly as you can or that they don't seem to care as much as you do—especially at work?

19. Would you say you're an adrenaline junkie?

20. Do people bore you?

21. Once you begin to stabilize your mood, either through pharmaceuticals or through emotional discipline, do you

often feel guilty about things you've done in the past to other people or to yourself?

22. When you are with family members and you are eating, would you rather just get on with eating and then go and sit down and visit, or would you like to continue to visit over dinner and then at the table afterward?

23. Do you ever have problems with self-hatred or not really being happy with who you are?

24. Do you wish you were somebody else?

25. Do you think other people have fewer problems than you do, not including people with terminal illnesses, but just people in everyday living situations?

Bipolar Checklist

Put a checkmark next to the items that apply to you. This is a simple test to help you and your doctor determine if you have symptoms consistent with bipolar or cycling depression.

_____ Have you ever felt so easily angered that you shouted at people or started fights more easily than usual?

_____ Has there ever been a time period when people told you that you didn't seem like your normal self? At this time, did you feel good and perhaps even hyper, or were you so hyper that you got into trouble?

_____ Have there ever been times when you felt more certain of yourself that usual?

_____ Have there been periods of time when you got less sleep than usual and didn't miss the sleep?

_____ Have you ever experienced periods of time when you talked more or your speech was faster or more pressured than usual?

_____ Have you ever had racing thoughts or intrusive thoughts that you couldn't get out of your head?

_____ Were there times in your life when you found it difficult to concentrate because you were so easily distracted?

_____ Have you had periods where you experienced more energy than usual and were able to complete more tasks, even though they may not have been as accurate as usual?

_____ Have you ever had times when you were more social than usual; for example, have you phoned friends in the middle of the night?

_____ Were there times in your life when you were much more interested in sex than usual?

_____ Have you had periods when you did things that were unusual for you or that others thought were extremely foolish or risky?

_____ Were there times when you spent too much money and got yourself and/or your family into financial trouble?

_____ If you checked yes to several questions, have many of these items occurred during the same period of time?

_____ Did these things cause you problems with being able to work, legal problems, relationship difficulties, or financial ruin?

The two above questionnaires are for your information only. If you answered yes to more than half the questions and are wondering if you could have bipolar disorder, please discuss it further with your health care provider.

BIBLIOGRAPHY

Amen M.D, Daniel. *Change Your Brain, Change Your Life*. New York: Three Rivers Press, 1999.

Comings M.D., David. *Tourette Syndrome and Human Behavior*. Toronto: Hope Press, 1990.

Hallowell M.D. Edward and John Ratey, M.D., *Driven to Distraction*. New York: Touchstone, 1995.

Papolos M.D. Demitri and Janice Papolos, *The Bipolar Child*. New York: Broadway. 2007.

Steele, Danielle. *His Bright Light*. New York: Delta, 2000.

KEITH CONRAD Five years later: As I re-read Turning Black and White Into Gray, I realize that this was the darkest point in my life. I often felt completely helpless, frightened, and pretty much ready to give up.

In starting treatment with therapy and medication, I began to understand that awareness allows choices. I began to see choices. I realized I had the choice to run my life, not let my life run me. THINK ABOUT IT! Are you running your life or is your life running you? Oh yes! You may say, "That's easy for you to say. You are not in my situation." No, I am not you, but I really think that I have felt the same pain and despair you have. Yes, you have a mood disorder! Yes, you also have choices. When I began looking at choices rather than negative thinking, things began to come together. NOT OVERNIGHT, but I will say I am happier, healthier, both physically and mentally, because I finally sat down, reviewed choices and acted upon them. Now I am not talking about positive thinking. You can think positively and the bill collectors will still take your furniture. No! Look at choices. If something doesn't work, you have the choice to try something else.

I tried seven different types of medication before I found what works for me. I tried four different therapists and learned different choices from each one. You can truly find PEACE. When I began to be calm, my intellect could function, I was able to control my addictions, finances, relationships and everything else. You begin to become AWARE! Aware that maybe your so-called friends are toxic, your job or business that makes you sick can be walked away from, and you have the choice to do something ten times more profitable that you enjoy. All of this sounds very prep-talk to you right now, but don't get me wrong. It worked for me and it can work for you, if you allow awareness, choices, and peace to work for you.

CHOICES:

Medication: Learning how you are supposed to feel is important. I had windows of time that certain meds let me feel calm and aware for the first time. Even when things didn't work permanently with that medication, I remembered the good feeling and had the choice to find other ways to hold on to it. Sometimes that was exercise, therapy, relaxation, or spending more time outdoors. Sometimes it was another medication. Being aware of the good feeling helped me make the changes in my life to find it again.

Therapy: Different methods helped. Becoming AWARE helped me make choices. EMDR helped me see both sides of the coin. Hypnotherapy helped me relax. It's all about awareness and choices.

Work: I spent 33 years in a trade I hated. The choice was to change my occupation and work on something more enjoyable. At first, this was financially terrifying, but now the money is coming in and I am happy.

Attitude: Stop negative thinking! It's a habit. When you get a negative mood or thought, make the choice not to let it run you. I don't mean saying, "I am going to replace this with love or positive thinking." Simply become aware of your thoughts so you can gradually learn to stop the negative ones. !

Peace or Insanity: I like this anonymous quote: "Peace does not mean to be in a place where there is no more trouble or hard work, it means to be in the midst of those things and be calm in your heart."

Run Your Life: It's your life. It may suck right now, but when I realized I was letting other people make me miserable, I made changes. This doesn't mean living like a hermit and giving up on your friends, spouse, co-workers, etc. It's giving yourself permission to let them know they are hurting you. What they do with it is their problem.

ARE YOU RUNNING YOUR LIFE OR IS YOUR LIFE RUNNING YOU?